DR. Yoga

NIRMALA HERIZA

Hatha Yoga Cardiac Therapist, Cedars-Sinai Medical Center

Preventive and Rehabilitative Cardiac Center

DR. *Yoga*

Yoga for Health

JEREMY P. TARCHER/PENGUIN

A MEMBER OF PENGUIN GROUP (USA) INC.

NEW YORK

W

The Hatha yoga postures given in this book are based on the Integral Yoga® method of Hatha Yoga instruction as taught by H.H. Sri Swami Satchidananda, as adapted by the author for use in her specialized practice. Any changes and adaptations from the original have been made solely by the author.

Integral Yoga® is a registered service mark of Satchidananda Ashram—Yogaville. Used with permission. All rights expressly reserved by Satchidananda Ashram—Yogaville.

Most Tarcher/Penguin books are available at special quantity discounts for bulk purchase for sales promotions, premiums, fundraising, and educational needs. Special books or book excerpts also can be created to fit specific needs. For details, write Penguin Group (USA) Inc. Special Markets, 375 Hudson Street, New York, NY 10014.

Every effort has been made to ensure that the information contained in this book is complete and accurate. However, neither the publisher nor the author is engaged in rendering professional advice or services to the individual reader. The ideas, procedures, and suggestions contained in this book are not intended as a substitute for consulting with your physician. All matters regarding your health require medical supervision. Neither the author nor the publisher shall be liable or responsible for any loss or damage allegedly arising from any information or suggestion in this book.

The recipes contained in this book are to be followed exactly as written. The publisher is not responsible for your specific health or allergy needs that may require medical supervision. The publisher is not responsible for any adverse reactions to the recipes contained in this book.

Jeremy P. Tarcher/Penguin
a member of
Penguin Group (USA) Inc.
375 Hudson Street
New York, NY 10014
www.penguin.com

Quotations from the works of Sri Swami Satchidananda used by permission of Satchidananda Ashram—Yogaville, copyright holder
Integral Yoga Hatha © 1970 Satchidananda Ashram—Yogaville
Key to Peace © 1976, 1989 Satchidananda Ashram—Yogaville
To Know Your Self: The Essential Teachings of Swami Satchidananda © 1978 Satchidananda Ashram—Yogaville
Cover photograph of the author: Art Streiber/Montage Photographic, Inc.

Library of Congress Cataloging-in-Publication Data

Heriza, Nirmala, date.
    Dr. Yoga : yoga for health / Nirmala Heriza.
      p.   cm.
    Includes bibliographical references.
    ISBN 1-58542-292-4
    1. Yoga, Hatha.   2. Health.   3. Exercise.   I. Title: Doctor Yoga.   II. Title.
    RA781.7.H466   2004   2004043545
    613.7'046—dc22

Printed in the United States of America
10   9   8   7   6   5   4   3   2   1

This book is printed on acid-free paper. ∞

Book design by Meighan Cavanaugh

In honor of my beloved guru,

H.H. Sri Swami Satchidananda Maharaj,

and the sacred science of yoga

This book is respectfully and gratefully dedicated to my guru, the world-renowned yoga master H.H. Sri Swami Satchidananda Maharaj, founder of the Integral Yoga Institutes and Ashrams, International. His Integral Yoga teachings provide the theoretical foundation for my work as a Hatha yoga cardiac specialist at Cedars-Sinai Medical Center. I also wish to respectfully acknowledge his guru, H.H. Sri Swami Sivananda Maharaj, H.H. Sri Patanjali, and all of the great spiritual masters throughout the ages, whose lives and teachings continue to contribute to the legacy of the sacred science of yoga.

Contents

Part One: Prevention

THE YOGA VITAMIN: A 10-MINUTE "HEAD-TO-TOE" MICRO-SESSION

Part Two: Rehabilitation

YOGA FOR HEALTH PRACTICE SET II: A RESTORATIVE YOGA PROGRAM FOR THE TREATMENT OF ACUTE AND CHRONIC DISEASE

MEDICAL MODELS

COMMON AILMENTS

Part Three: Nutrition

by Mary Felando, M.S., R.D., Cardiovascular Nutrition Specialist for the
Preventive and Rehabilitative Cardiac Center at Cedars-Sinai Medical Center

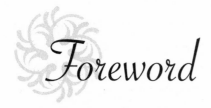

Foreword

I first met Nirmala Heriza in 1972, more than thirty years ago, in Santa Barbara when she was coleading the first Integral Yoga retreat that I attended with the legendary ecumenical teacher Sri Swami Satchidananda. Even then, her intelligence, passion for yoga, and charismatic eloquence helped inspire me to begin practicing yoga and meditation. It was a life-transforming experience for me.

As I began to experience the benefits in my own life, my colleagues and I at the non-profit Preventive Medicine Research Institute began to document the power of yoga and meditation in health and healing. We were able to demonstrate, for the first time, in a series of randomized controlled trials, that the progression of even severe heart disease often could begin to reverse when people began making comprehensive lifestyle changes. These included the regular practice of yoga and meditation, changes in diet (to predominantly low-fat, plant-based whole foods), moderate exercise, and support groups. These research findings were published in peer-reviewed medical journals, including the *Journal of the American Medical Association, The Lancet, Circulation, The New England Journal of Medicine, The American Journal of Cardiology,* and others.

In subsequent demonstration projects, we found that these changes were not only medically effective but also cost-effective. In brief, we found that almost 80 percent of people who were eligible for bypass surgery or angioplasty were able to avoid it safely by making these comprehensive lifestyle changes. Mutual of Omaha calculated an immediate savings of almost $30,000 per patient. These patients reported reductions in angina comparable to what can be achieved with bypass surgery or angioplasty without the costs or risks of surgery. These findings were published in the *American Journal of Cardiology* in November 1998. We also found that patients who needed bypass surgery or angioplasty were able to reduce the likelihood of needing another operation by making comprehensive lifestyle changes after surgery. Medicare is now conducting a demonstration project in which they are paying for 1,800 patients to go through this program at sites my colleagues and I have trained.

Thus, yoga has come a long way in the past twenty-five years. When I began our first study in 1977, one of the cardiologists took me aside and said, "Dean, I can't refer my patients to a study in which you're teaching people yoga and meditation. What am I going to say, that I'm referring them to a swami?" So we called it "stress management techniques" instead of yoga, even though most stress management techniques really derive from yoga.

Now, yoga is on the cover of *Time* magazine and has become a household word. While there are many yoga teachers, there are very few with the experience, integrity, and training of Nirmala Heriza. She brings a level of professionalism as well as joy that are tremendously inspiring.

Nirmala has played an important role in bringing yoga into the mainstream of modern medicine. She has taught yoga and meditation to cardiac patients at Cedars-Sinai Medical Center in Los Angeles as well as to others around the world. As president of the United Council on Yoga and a copartner of the President's Council on Physical Fitness and Sports, she carries this even further.

This book is a manifestation of the best of her work and is a wonderful guide for both preventing the most common diseases and as an adjunct treatment to conventional medicine for those who need it. It will be a great service to so many people.

—DEAN ORNISH, M.D.
Founder and President, Preventive Medicine Research Institute
Clinical Professor of Medicine, University of California, San Francisco
Author *Dr. Dean Ornish's Program for Reversing Heart Disease* and *Love and Survival*

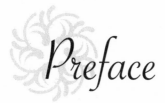

Preface

The use of yoga as a stress management technique has gained importance and credence, especially over the last ten years. It is now widely used and accepted by the lay public, especially those who realize the benefits that yoga provides to them in their daily lives. For some, the word *yoga* itself summons thoughts of being too "weird" or "eclectic," but now yoga is seen as one of the leading preventive health ideas in the area of stress reduction, health, and well-being, and is being used in the realm of cardiovascular disease as a part of therapy. In the scientific community it has taken a long period of time to gain acceptance for the use of yoga as a stress management therapy. In the mid-seventies, researchers around the world began to show how effective stress management techniques could be. They were proving that meditation, progressive relaxation, and visual imagery could lower blood pressure and reduce cholesterol levels. Most of these meditation techniques derive from yoga. The use of all these yoga techniques can become a very powerful tool for stress management. Yoga should be seen as a complement to our approach to medical care. At the Preventive and Rehabilitative Cardiac Center in Los Angeles, the program uses a style of Hatha yoga as taught by our Hatha yoga cardiac therapist, Nirmala Heriza, with its patient population as one of its main therapies for stress management. With our knowledge of how stress can have detrimental effects on individuals, especially in the area of coronary disease, we decided more than ten years ago to begin using yoga with our patients. It has been well received by the cardiac rehabilitation patient population.

—C. Noel Bairey Merz, M.D.
Director of Cedars-Sinai Medical Center Preventive and Rehabilitative Cardiac Center

with Richard Gordon, M.A.

Introduction

The Vision

On June 23, 2002, the United States of America made a quantum leap in its official position on healthcare. Dr. Tommy Thompson, director of the U.S. Department of Health and Human Services, announced that "the direction of healthcare in America will now officially be 'prevention.'" This announcement was made before a panel of distinguished physicians during the live telecast of the Summit on Health Forum, on the MSNBC network, hosted by Brian Williams. It followed President Bush's press conference in which he made physical activity and fitness a central cornerstone of his administration.

Like never before, we in the West are involved in a medical and health revolution, a dynamic, world-changing revolution in which Eastern and Western medical ideologies are converging and being reorganized into a new system of "vertical integration." Acupuncture is meeting the hypodermic needle. Pharmaceuticals, surgery and other Western medical approaches to treating physical illness are collaborating with and at times completely deferring to Eastern therapeutic protocols such as yoga, which, as just one example, was clinically proven by Dr. Dean Ornish to help both prevent and reverse heart disease.

Over the past decade, I have had the distinct privilege of being strategically involved in the process of integrating Eastern and Western modalities into the medical mainstream, while serving as Hatha yoga cardiac therapist for Cedars-Sinai Medical Center Preventive and Rehabilitative Cardiac Center in Los Angeles, California. As part of the esteemed team of medical experts who staff the Cedars-Sinai cardiology department, including the eminent P. K. Shah, M.D., Dr. C. Noel Bairey Merz and Dr. Donna Polk, as well as medical directors and the patient and program coordinator, Richard Gordon, M.A., I conduct classes and consult privately with both acute- and chronic-care patients who are assimilating yoga and nutrition into their conventional medical protocols.

I also network with well-known physicians in their specialties, including Dean Ornish, M.D., the famed cardiac specialist who medically pioneered the critically acclaimed program for reversing heart disease through yoga and diet, based on Sri Swami Satchidananda's Teachings of Integral Yoga, and Sandra McLanahan, M.D., coauthor of the groundbreaking book *Surgery and Its Alternatives,* who provides expert medical commentary for this book.

In November 2001, due to the recognition my work at Cedars-Sinai Medical Center received in the May 2001 issue of *Time* magazine, I was contacted by a representative from the President's Council on Fitness and Sports in Washington, D.C., and invited to participate in its physical activity and fitness programs as a representative of yoga.

Subsequently, the United Council on Yoga was formed with the guidance of world-renowned yoga master and founder of Integral Yoga International, Sri Swami Satchidananda. The council's associations and governing membership include Cedars-Sinai Medical Center, Dean Ornish's Preventive Medicine Institute, the Integral Yoga Institute, and various eminent medical and yoga dignitaries throughout the world.

In 2003 the United Council on Yoga was invited to be an official cosponsor with the President's Challenge Programs under the umbrella of the President's Council on Fitness and Sports to help support and implement the nation's physical activity programs, with yoga as a central focus.

In my official capacity as president of the United Council on Yoga, I have had the privilege and unique opportunity over the past year of collaborating with Marine Commander Penny Royall (former executive director of the President's Council on Fitness and Sports), Melissa Johnson (executive director of the President's Council on Fitness and Sports), Christine Spain (director of the President's Challenge Programs) and other Washington dignitaries in this groundbreaking and exciting new direction for health and fitness. The opportunity to play a pivotal role in this historic and unprecedented effort to endorse and encourage physical activity and preventive healthcare, and to inform my readers of the vast potential of available natural resources for recovery and rehabilitation, have provided the inspiration for the vision and served as a vital launchpad for this book.

My Personal Journey

How Yoga Saved My Life

In the early 1970s I was living in New York City and working in Off-Broadway productions, experimental theater and music. I had been briefly introduced to Hatha yoga *asanas* (physical postures) by guest playwright/director Megan Terry when I was an undergraduate majoring in theater arts and communications at Immaculate Heart College in Los Angeles, but had drifted away from the practice.

At the time, my diet consisted mainly of fried, fatty and carbohydrate-intensive foods, supplemented by tons of caffeine and a three-pack-a-day cigarette habit—a cardiologist's nightmare. A heart attack waiting to happen. And I was only twenty. With my immune system (the body's "tactical defense force") compromised to the max and suffering from oxygen deprivation, I developed chronic bronchitis, a debilitating respiratory condition, and I had to rely on regular courses of penicillin to stay alive. While my creative energy was charged and optimized, physically I was at ground zero.

The dedicated physician who kept reviving me medically from my raging episodes of bronchitis gave me shocking admonitions about the risk of having even one more cigarette. I was in that place of desperate solitude with my addiction, knowing I needed to quit but not having the strength or willpower to try. In those days, before nicotine gum or patches were available, I was faced with going cold turkey. That was impossible to imagine.

"How will I hold a conversation?" I would ask myself. "What will I do with my hands?" While nicotine is certainly not as nefarious an addiction as some, as with all addictions, quitting can become a perilous self-perpetuating cycle. I was a hamster in a wheel. Considering the ultimatum made me smoke all the more. I was nearing the precipice of despair when my good friend, actress Sally Kirkland, came to my rescue. In her customary take-no-prisoners manner, she convinced me that I needed to do yoga. It had saved her life, many times. And it would save mine. Skeptical that something as simple as yoga could be the answer to the complexity of my problems, I grabbed my Winstons and headed uptown the next day to the Integral Yoga Institute on West End Avenue, where Sally conducted classes. That's where I first found out about Sri Swami Satchidananda's teachings of Integral Yoga.

Swamiji offered encouragement to anyone in the death grip of addiction. According to him, a person who regularly practices yoga will automatically lose the desire for the abusive substance—no matter what it is. He spoke from experience: He himself had been a heavy smoker.

Three times a week, without fail, I began taking Hatha yoga classes. Incrementally, I started feeling stronger and healthier, until, after approximately two and a half months, to my surprise, the seductive need for cigarettes grew less and less, and I started leaving them behind in my apartment when I traveled uptown to my classes. My lungs craved oxygen more than the dense gray smoke that had filled them, and I actually became repelled by the thought of having a cigarette.

Raja Yoga

Swami Satchidananda was right. According to a philosophy of yoga (*Raja yoga*), the discipline I was engaged in is referred to as *pratipaksha bhavana*. This practice consists of replacing a negative substance or thought with a positive one. Eventually the positive one wins out. You can do the same with your mind, or with an emotion such as anger. When you're in its grasp, mentally step back from it and view it from an objective vantage point. Then supplant it with a pleasant, inspiring thought.

Think of a place or person you love, or whatever inspires you. Keep doing that and eventually the anger will dissipate. If you need to analyze the cause of the anger, you can designate time to do that later. In the meantime, this simple practice diffuses the emotion.

The more you practice this technique, the easier it becomes. Many modern-day psychologists use this technique with their patients. Dr. Ornish recommends it in his Program for Reversing Heart Disease, and I use it effectively with many of my cardiac patients today.

Like many students new to the practice, I thought at first that yoga was limited to the physical postures ("Hatha yoga"). Gradually I learned that yoga is a *complete* science, or a synthesis of practices—the poses (*asanas*), meditation, self-analysis, nutrition, self-awareness—that, when combined, influence and inform not just our physical but also our mental, emotional and spiritual health. In this way, you can create total health.

At Swamiji's suggestion I gradually went a step further and stopped eating meat and all of its relatives, such as eggs. I began a "yoga friendly" or lacto-vegetarian diet (see page 211) that allowed dairy products and offered many meat-free alternatives for protein.

Integral Yoga, or the synthesis of yoga disciplines, was my launchpad for recovery from a debilitating chronic illness that had lain dormant in my system, like Darth Vader and the storm troopers, ready to strike at the first sign of weakness. The recovery process from addiction, as anyone trapped in one will tell you, takes time and patience, and unyielding vigilence. At times it can seem impossible. It's bleak and lonely. And there is always a voice out there, somewhere in the wind, calling your name and eager to draw you back in.

My recovery also meant finding a way to rebuild my immune system and to stop relying on the penicillin antibiotic that had become my messiah. This was harder than it seemed. It was a different kind of addiction—a more sophisticated kind that pharmaceutical company marketing executives lie awake at night dreaming about.

In the mid-1970s I returned to the warmer temperatures of California, where I eventually became a certified full-time yoga instructor and executive director of the Integral Yoga Institute in San Francisco. Teaching Yoga deepened my own practice. I'm not one of those people who experience a "galactic" light show or supernatural phenomena in my meditations, no matter how long and unremittingly I practice. And when I do Hatha yoga, I'm still not able to lock my legs into a 180-degree position behind my head like my guru or Madonna. However, as all the enlightened exponents of yoga and meditation will tell you, the "special effects" or advanced multiple-jointed asana positions, while nice, are just the icing. The real reward is the benefit you receive from dedicated practice every day. The "super achievements and experiences" can actually hinder or distract you from the ultimate goal—a calm and steady mind and a body of perfect health. For me, the crowning achievement was finally controlling my addiction to nicotine and recovering from chronic respiratory disease. Even though, after so many years, I still want a cigarette once in a while, through the daily practice of yoga I have the strength to resist.

A Medical Approach

In 1980 I left San Francisco to become director of the Integral Yoga Center in Los Angeles. Inspired by the role that alternative medicine practices such as acupuncture, acupressure and homeopathy had played in my recovery, I began postgraduate studies in Oriental medicine and eventually became certified in the Jin Shin Ryho system of acupressure. In this system, pressure is applied simultaneously to combined points (tsubos) on the various meridians to increase energy flow to specific organs.

I interned with David Kearney, O.M.D., acupuncture specialist to Hollywood's film and music celebrity community, and gradually developed my own private practice, combining yoga with these Oriental medical techniques. My celebrity clientele read like a Who's Who: Candice Bergen, Jane Fonda, George Harrison, Lindsay Crouse, Oliver Stone, Diane Ladd, Moon Zappa, Laura Dern and many others, all of whom were turning their attention to alternative medicine and to the importance of a more natural way of keeping themselves spiritually and emotionally focused and physically healthy.

At the peak of this activity I became the exclusive Integral Yoga instructor for the legendary Jane Fonda Workout Program, in a shocking turnabout from the program's usual lineup of aerobics, powerstairs and weight-training classes. The floors pulsated to the driving rhythms of Madonna and Michael Jackson, played at window-shattering decibels, while in well-polished studio B, my students were quietly getting healthy and high on yoga.

To my constant amazement as a clinical practitioner, I repeatedly observed the profound therapeutic effects of yoga as an adjunct therapy for acute and chronic disease. I saw miracles happen. One patient in particular continues to confound her physicians. And me. Within a span of five years, Buffy Stewart, a well-known folk singer, writer and dancer, was diagnosed with a complicated benign brain tumor and colon cancer. Combining yoga with her conventional clinical protocols, she recovered from both pathologies and today leads a normal, healthy, physically active life. Her neurosurgeon told her he had never seen anyone with her particular diagnosis make such a dramatic recovery. Her oncologist said the complete absence of cancer in Buffy's body was, in her clinical experience, unprecedented.

The Beginning of a Beautiful Friendship

In 1992 I received a call from renowned cardiologist C. Noel Bairey Merz, M.D., medical director of Cedars-Sinai Medical Center Preventive and Rehabilitative Cardiac Center in Beverly Hills. I had been recommended by Dean Ornish, M.D., the respected cardiac specialist who shot to fame with his best-selling book *Program for Reversing Heart Disease,* based on his groundbreaking theories using yoga as a primary modality for preventing, treating and reversing heart disease. Because of my medical background and training in Integral Yoga with Swami Satchidananda, I had been invited by Dr. Ornish to serve as his Los Angeles–based yoga therapist referral consultant. Clinically, it was the Integral Yoga teachings of Swami Satchidananda that provided the theory, substance and paradigm for Dr. Ornish's program. Inspired by the results of his research, Dr. Merz was seeking a yoga therapist trained in the same effective tradition of yoga that was the basis of Dr. Ornish's program to become part of the cardiac program at Cedars.

> *A body of perfect health, and strength, mind with all clarity and calmness. Intellect as sharp as a razor, Will as pliable as steel. Heart full of love and compassion. Life full of dedication and Realization of the True Self is the Goal of Yoga.*
>
> —Sri Swami Satchidananda

I was profoundly honored by this prestigious invitation. I accepted his invitation and developed a therapeutic program for Cedars-Sinai that was based on the Integral Yoga® method of Hatha yoga instruction as taught by Sri Swami Satchidananda. I was also inspired and impressed by Dr. Merz's courage in integrating into her work at a major mainstream hospital a discipline still being scrutinized by many in the medical establishment.

Those of us who have the privilege of being a part of this historical new collaboration of Western medicine and yoga are witness to a beautiful new friendship that will continue to reform the face of healthcare in the twenty-first century and beyond.

How to Use This Book

The best way to approach *Dr. Yoga*'s Yoga for Health program is as your own personal yoga health therapist. A step-by-step companion and tool, this book will guide you through preventing and treating a range of conditions as well as promote general good health. However, if you have been diagnosed with a condition or disease, you should consult your physician before beginning the Yoga for Health program.

This book is organized into three sections: Prevention, Rehabilitation and Nutrition. I strongly recommend that you read it from cover to cover to familiarize yourself with the fundamentals of yoga and the specific principles of using yoga as a tool for preventing and treating disease. It will answer your questions and enable you to derive a more comprehensive and complete benefit.

Part One

Part I consists of an easy-to-follow beginner-level Yoga for Health program of asanas and practices based on the Integral Yoga® system of Hatha yoga. This Yoga for Health program has been clinically verified to prevent disease. The instructional text describes the specific therapeutic value of each *asana* (posture). This complete Yoga for Health program serves as the fundamental holistic basis for the poses targeted at specific health conditions that follow.

A unique and vital signature feature of Part I is this program of asanas. By design, this section breaks down the anatomy into distinct physical systems and identifies diseases that are common to each system. You can use this section to reinforce areas where you might be vulnerable. For example, if you have a predisposition to head and chest colds, you might want to pay particular attention to your lungs and the organs that support your immune system. If you are a woman suffering from regular debilitating episodes of PMS or menstrual cramps, or are either pre-menopausal or menopausal, you might want to do postures that promote circulation to the ovaries and uterus and that support the central nervous system.

The head-to-toe asanas in this section are postures you can do each day as an adjunct to the complete Yoga for Health program, to strengthen and enhance the health of a particular system and thus prevent disease.

Micro-Session

The micro-session is a ten-minute program of distilled Yoga for Health Hatha poses for the time-challenged homemaker, executive, working professional or student, perfectly designed to fit into a busy and hectic schedule so there is never an excuse not to do your Hatha yoga practice. You can do it anytime. Anywhere. Just take that mid-morning or -afternoon break and make it happen.

This program specifically strengthens both the immune and the cardiovascular systems, and is engineered to help you get through a full-throttle stressful day—the kind of day that, in time, breaks down your immune and nervous systems until you end up in the doctor's office or in bed. The kind of day that contributes to the aging process. The micro-session is also presented with a photo-illustrated practice guide of postures with an emphasis on the particular organs that generally regulate circulation and manage stress. Instructional text details how to do each asana and describes its specific medical benefits.

CAVEAT: Under no circumstances should the physical systems or micro-session adjuncts be construed as a substitute for the complete Yoga for Health program. As I've mentioned, and as any physician will tell you, there are no shortcuts to health. Yoga is a holistic science, and there is a fundamental logic at work behind the sequence of poses and practices utilized in the program as a whole. In order to be assured of the optimal benefit, the practitioner needs to adhere regularly to the complete program, at least three times a week. Otherwise it would be akin to isolating one or two supplements such as calcium and magnesium to do the work of the full spectrum of vitamins and minerals the body requires for maximum natural health. Ultimately, this would of course be counterproductive and wouldn't make sense.

Part Two

Rehabilitation is specifically dedicated to the treatment of acute and chronic disease. It is strategically divided according to condition/disease and includes physician/patient testimonies along with specific clinical recommendations for using Hatha yoga as part of your treatment program. The clinical studies have been carefully documented by a diverse network of eminent physicians, professional healthcare providers and medical authorities throughout the world.

The physician/patient studies serve a twofold purpose. First, they demonstrate how yoga is being taken seriously as a form of treatment and is breaking new ground in the medical mainstream among physicians and conventional medical institutions. Second, they provide you the reader with the personal experiences of patients who have been diagnosed with a life-threatening or debilitating disease and have made a full recovery and returned to a normal and functional lifestyle. I hope these testimonies answer questions you or someone you care for might have, and dispel common misconceptions or fears about yoga as a reliable method of treatment and recovery. I am confident these personal stories will help open your world to the potential of this age-old science.

Like Part I, Part II includes an illustrated guide, instructional text and a description of the medical benefits of each of the restorative Hatha yoga poses. This is the therapeutic program I use with my patients in the Cedars-Sinai Preventive and Rehabilitative Hatha Yoga Cardiac Program and the basic protocol that Dr. Ornish recommends in his program for reversing heart disease. Although as a restorative program it has been clinically determined to be effective in the treatment of heart disease, the same sequence of modified poses is also used in the treatment of other conditions such as cancer, arthritis, chronic fatigue and respiratory disease as well as addiction problems and neuromuscular and musculoskeletal disorders.

As I mentioned earlier, if you have been diagnosed with a particular condition or disease and are planning to use the restorative Yoga for Health program as a therapeutic adjunct to your physician's conventional treatment plan for your physical rehabilitation, contact either a professional health practitioner trained in Integral Yoga Hatha or a professional yoga therapist versed in the basic principles of nonstrenuous therapeutic Hatha yoga, to work with you and your physician in your therapeutic regime. If you choose to embark upon the restorative Yoga for Health program on your own, without the direction of a clinical yoga therapist, consult with your physician and use it only under medical supervision.

If you are seeking a physician, healthcare provider or clinical yoga therapist to consult with for treatment, see Resources (page 267) for a comprehensive, reliable list of medical and therapeutic yoga professionals and medical facilities that include yoga as a treatment protocol.

Part Three

Part III includes a yoga-friendly, vegetarian-based nutritional guide that provides the scientific basis and rationale for a healthy vegetarian diet designed by Mary Felando, M.A., licensed dietitian and nutritionist for Cedars-Sinai Medical Center Preventive and Rehabilitative Cardiac Center. Her program, created uniquely for this book, includes a two-week-long, easy-to-prepare sample menu as well as healthful recipes.

I look forward to taking you on both a personal and a practical journey through a medically verified system of yoga, providing you with not only a practical self-help guide but also medical case studies and testimonies by people from all walks of life with firsthand experience of the physiological and psychological benefits of yoga. Throughout this book you will read the words of people who have used yoga not only to optimize their health and well-being but also to recover from such diseases and conditions as cancer, diabetes, depression, arthritis, memory loss and addiction. My ultimate goal is to provide you with a comprehensive, diverse and practical manual on yoga that will serve as a constant companion to both your everyday health needs and more serious medical conditions—one that will dispel misconceptions and instill confidence in this profound, ancient science designed to provide us all with a longer, healthier and more dynamic life.

To quote my inimitable yoga master, Sri Swami Satchidananda, "Health is your birthright, not disease."

A Brief History of Yoga

There are diverse theories as to when and how yoga originated. The general consensus among pundits is that it was somewhere between 300 B.C. and A.D. 5,000, which gives it a significant head start over most scientific endeavors.

By definition, yoga is a composite of principles and practices designed to integrate and promote the developmental health of the body and mind. While yoga is a science and not a religion, ultimately it is meant to unite the individual with the spirit or life force that sustains the universe. In a few simple words, yoga is designed to make us healthy, happy and peaceful and to optimize every aspect of our lives. The philosophy and practices of yoga that have been proven to restore health and expand the consciousness of the mind have a very practical, reality-based application. They're where the rubber of the philosophy meets the road.

The renowned Indian sage Bhagavan Patanjali Maharishi originally organized the various elements of the yoga science into an eight-step system commonly referred to as ashtanga yoga. Inspired by Patanjali, there are several distinguished traditions of yoga taught today that have been developed by enlightened and renowned yoga masters or gurus throughout the centuries. My guru, Sri Swami Satchidananda, has formulated a synthesis of yoga into what he calls Integral Yoga. It's a complete, scientifically based, physician-verified program of health for life that serves as the philosophical and practical basis for this book.

Integral Yoga, as a system, includes the following practices:

- Raja Yoga: The path of concentration and meditaion.
- Japa Yoga: The concentrated repetition of a mantra (a sound vibration representing an aspect of the Divine).
- Hatha Yoga: Postures (asanas), breath control (pranayama), and relaxation.
- Karma Yoga: The path of selfless service without attachment to the fruits of one's action.
- Bhakti Yoga: The path of love and devotion to God or a higher power.
- Jnana Yoga: The path of wisdom through self-analysis and awareness.

The Hatha yoga program featured in this book is based on the non-strenuous, easy-to-do Integral Yoga Hatha method I use in a clinical setting at Cedars-Sinai Medical Center, and used by Dr. Ornish.

What Is Hatha Yoga?

Hatha yoga, or the "physical aspect," is the beginning step in the synthesis of yoga. It includes a science of bodily postures (*asanas*), deep relaxation, breath control (*pranayama*), cleansing processes (*kriyas*) and mental concentration techniques. In the system of Hatha yoga, the asanas are non-strenuous stretches that increase flexibility and tone and strengthen the musculature, stabilize and balance the nervous system and promote circulation in all major organs and glands. The practices also help to promote psychological equanimity. The regular performance of the combined Hatha yoga postures and practices has been clinically observed by medical practitioners throughout the world to enhance overall health and both prevent and reverse disease. Yoga is often referred to as "the fountain of youth" because there is clinical evidence that it slows the aging process and promotes long life. Symptoms of aging, such as wrinkles and a poor complexion, are caused by poor circulation of the blood, allowing metabolic waste products or toxins to build up in the system. Through the practice of the yoga asanas, blood circulation is restored and the metabolic waste products are washed out, resulting in a more youthful look and feeling.

It is for these reasons that, as my book explains in detail, traditional Hatha yoga as a therapy is being utilized by physicians and healthcare practitioners such as Dr. Ornish, Dr. Sandra McLanahan, Dr. Mehmet Oz, Dr. Stephen Pacia and myself; and by medical institutions such as Cedars-Sinai Medical Center, New York Presbyterian Hospital and New York University Medical Center in the prevention and treatment of cardiovascular disease as well as other conditions such as asthma, diabetes, cancer, obesity, epilepsy, addiction and depression.

Misconceptions About Hatha Yoga

If You Do It Right, It Should Hurt

Patanjali defined a posture as an "easy pose," one that gives steadiness and comfort. Doing a posture, or asana, without strain or force eliminates the risk of injury. Because exercise implies quick movement and a degree of exertion or strain, Hatha yoga is more accurately understood to be a therapeutic stretching regime, not an exercise program. If you are injured doing yoga, it isn't really yoga.

Daily I encounter prospective Hatha yoga students who express apprehension about yoga. They tell me they either are intimidated by it or have tried it and gotten injured doing it. Some of the most popular excuses for not doing yoga are:

"It's too hard."

"I'm not thin enough. I'm too fat."

"I'm not flexible enough. I can't touch my knees, let alone my toes."

"I'm not healthy enough."

"My mind is too distracted."

"Frankly, I'm an A-type personality and it won't work for me."

"I'm too old."

"I sprained my ankle doing it once."

In the current yoga trend, many non-practitioners have been led to believe that yoga involves wrapping your legs around your head and 180-degree joint flexibility. Or that it is an aggressive and difficult activity. Many actually equate yoga with joint-defying feats of acrobatics, not unlike those performed by Cirque de Soleil. While it's true that there are advanced practitioners who are able to achieve extraordinary degrees of flexibility and perform gravity-defying feats—*Vanity Fair* and *Harper's Bazaar* magazines have featured exquisite famous examples—these levels of achievement, while stunning and exemplary, can take years to accomplish. Not everyone has the dance background, joint physiology and endurance to sustain that level of practice. Let alone the time. Which is why my guru emphasizes simplicity. The ultimate goal of yoga is to achieve a balanced, healthy body and a calm, focused mind, which anyone can attain. All the medical practitioners I work with would heartily agree. Simply stated, you do not need to be flexible, thin, focused, young or even healthy to do yoga. Yoga can help you attain those goals.

A-type personalities often make the best practitioners because they are highly motivated to succeed. In the case of yoga, success is measured by personal health standards. And yoga can help a person deal with the stresses of life. As an example, I had a stockbroker as a patient for many years whose blood systolic pressure, which is created by the initial contraction of the heart, stabilized from 170 to 120 because of his yoga practice.

No one is excluded. No matter your age or health, there are appropriate levels of yoga for every individual's ability. While the Hatha yoga components of this book are geared primarily to the beginning practitioner, everyone from the beginner to the most advanced practitioner can benefit from the medical information provided.

Throughout my many years of teaching Hatha yoga and using it as a clinical tool to treat acute and chronic disease, not one person who has approached me with an argument or apprehension about his or her ability to do Hatha yoga has been disappointed with the results.

Basic Guidelines for Beginning Your Practice of Hatha Yoga

Keep in mind that there are no quick fixes. The practice of yoga requires diligence, discipline and patience. The rewards, however, are great, and the benefits tangible and enduring. It's like finding gold at the end of the rainbow.

You do not need props, hanging ropes or exotic devices to perform a pose, although some methods recommend them. Most yoga masters, like mine, recommend keeping your practice simple. The Integral Yoga method requires no external or expensive accessories. You do not need mirrors. In fact, they can distract you from doing the postures. Yoga is generally done with the eyes closed to promote concentration. Focusing on a posture with your eyes closed enhances its benefits.

You don't need a formal class to do yoga. Although a group dynamic can be supportive, by tradition yoga is a solitary discipline that can be practiced anywhere. If possible, do your asanas in a quiet, comfortable place with a pleasant atmosphere where you won't be distracted. If this isn't possible, you can do it anywhere: at work, in a limited space—it's supremely adaptable to your individual needs and circumstances.

If you're on a hard surface, use a thick, natural-fiber mat or folded blanket for your poses. If you're on a soft carpet or rug, use a towel to lie on. Avoid uneven or slanted surfaces, drafty conditions and direct sunlight.

If you don't have a personal yoga instructor, use an instructional video or audiotape to accompany this instructional manual. There are a list of tapes and videos in Resources, such as "Yoga with a Master" by Swami Satchidananda, used by the active cardiac patients at Cedars-Sinai Medical Center.

Dietary Recommendations

Refrain from eating an hour before your practice. Drinking liquids is fine. However, avoid using alchohol or other stimulants such as caffeine.

While you certainly don't have to be a vegetarian to practice Hatha yoga, the nutritional segment of this book provides information about the health benefits of vegetarianism and provides extraordinary gourmet vegetarian recipes.

What to Wear

Loose, comfortable clothing made from natural fibers, which allow your body to breathe, are recommended. However, tights and leotards or shorts and a T-shirt can also be worn. What is most important is that you wear something that won't constrict or impede your movements or circulation and that will allow you to relax.

That said, I present this book as a medically verified system of health, vitality and fitness for all ages. I offer it as an easy-to-do program of prevention and rehabilitation for the skeptic and the cynic as well as for the believer. I offer it as an invitation for health for anyone with the desire to discover well-being and rejuvenation through the safe and clinically sound science of yoga.

PART One

Prevention

The Yoga for Health Practice Set that follows forms the groundwork for a yoga practice that supports and nurtures your health. Yoga is a holistic practice and, as such, requires that you never pay attention to one part of your body to the neglect of any other. The complete guide to nurturing a healthy body from head to toe contained in the remainder of this section is intended only as an adjunct to the Yoga for Health Program that follows. I urge you to do this thirty-minute practice set at least three times a week and to look upon it as the primary model and reference point for a truly healthful yoga practice.

Yoga for Health Practice Set I: A 30-Minute Program for Maintaining and Nurturing a Healthy Body and Mind

Beginning Level

CLASS TIME: 30 MINUTES

❋ ARDDHA PADMASANA (HALF LOTUS POSE) ❋

Sit with your legs stretched forward. Rest your right foot on your left thigh with the sole turned upward. Let your right knee touch the floor. Fold your left leg so that your left heel rests under your right thigh. Place your hands on your knees, palms up or down.

Clinical Benefits
This pose has been clinically noted to increase the output of blood from the heart, proving effective in the treatment of various forms of cardiovascular disease.

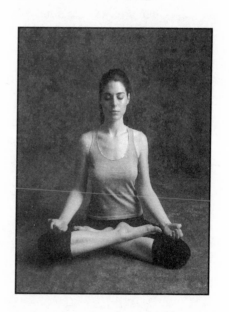

Beginning the Class

Chant the "om" syllable three times to create a peaceful sensation in your nervous system and mind. Inhale. The "o" emanates from the abdomen, releasing tension in the abdominal cavity, and rises through the chest. The "m" consonant resonates in the head, stimulating the production of the hormone serotonin, bringing forth a relaxed sensation in the mind and central nervous system.

❀ NETHRA VYAYAMAM (EYE EXERCISES) ❀

In performing the eye exercises that follow, remember to move slowly and with awareness. When your eyes are open, don't look at any particular object; simply focus on the natural movement of your eyes. Be careful not to strain. Center and close your eyes after each exercise.

1. Sitting in a cross-legged position, close your eyes and relax.
2. Open your eyes and move them from right to left four times.
3. Move your eyes up and down (from your forehead to your lap) four times.
4. Move your eyes in a clockwise rotation four times. Extend your gaze to the periphery.
5. Move your eyes in a counterclockwise rotation four times.
6. Bring your gaze back to the center and close your eyes.

Bring the palms of your hands together, brushing them back and forth until you create heat between them. Cup your palms over your eyes, allowing them to absorb the heat and energy from your hands, which helps to relax your eyes.

Clinical Benefits

These eye exercises help to relieve eye strain, tone the optic nerve and, in some cases, when practiced on a regular basis can improve vision.

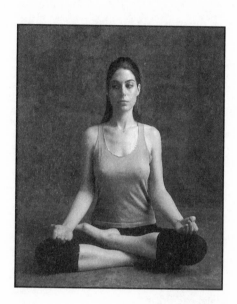

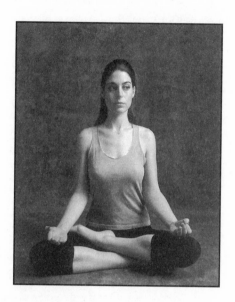

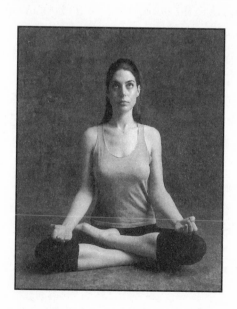

❧ SURYA NAMASKARAM (SUN SALUTATION) ❧

This is a series of twelve asanas (poses) done consecutively. One pose flows into the next in a smooth, dancelike fashion. There should be no strain involved.

1. Stand with your legs together. Bring your palms together at your chest.
2. Lock your thumbs and stretch your arms straight out in front of you, then up, bending back slightly at the pelvis. Look up at your hands.
3. Bend forward and drop over your legs, keeping your knees straight. Bring your head toward your knees. Unlock your thumbs and relax your spine and arms.
4. Place the palms of your hands on the floor beside your feet (it's all right to bend your knees for comfort). Stretch your left leg back, placing the knee on the floor. Look up.
5. Stretch your right leg back to meet the left and raise your buttocks so you form a triangle, with your head between your arms. Look back at your feet. Gently stretch your heels toward the floor.
6. Lower your knees to the floor. Bring your chest and chin to the floor. Your chest should be positioned between your hands.
7. Press your pelvis to the floor and curl your spine and head up, keeping your elbows slightly bent. Do not push or strain.
8. Rise into the triangle pose again, looking back at your feet.
9. Bring your left foot forward between your hands and place your right knee on the floor. Look up.
10. Bring the right leg forward to meet the left and relax over your straightened legs, looking back at your knees.
11. Lock your thumbs together again, palms open. Stretch your arms up and back alongside your ears. Press your pelvis back slightly. Look back at your hands.
12. Return to an erect position, palms together at your chest.

Relax with your arms alongside your body. Repeat three times.

Clinical Benefits

Stretches the entire body, increasing circulation into the heart, lungs and all the major organs, muscles and joints. It tones all the major muscle groups and promotes spinal flexibility, rejuvenating the nervous system. It stimulates the endocrine system, helping to support the immune function. It is beneficial in the prevention and treatment of arthritis by promoting the secretion of synovial fluid in the joints.

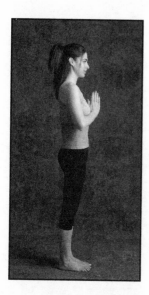
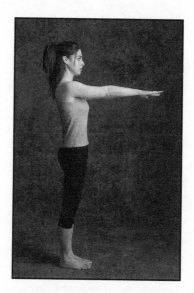
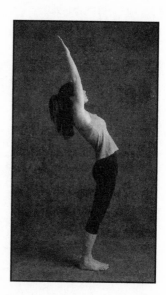

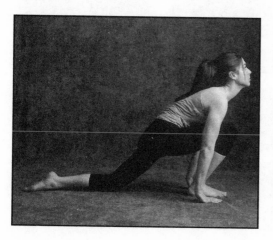
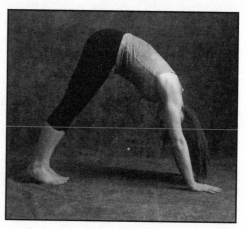

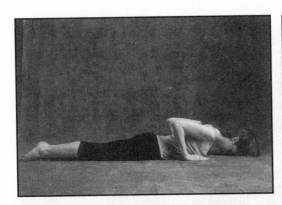

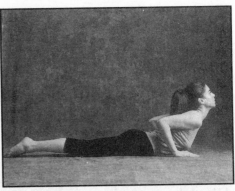

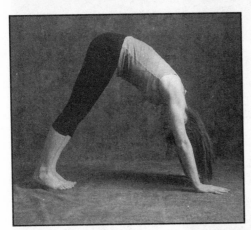

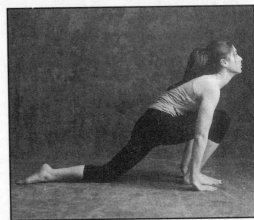

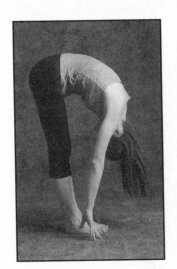

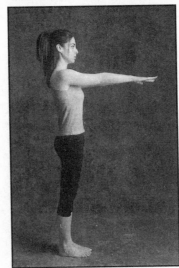

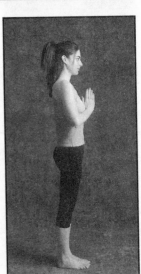

❈ SAVASANA (RELAXATION POSE) ❈

Lie on your back with your arms and legs extended and your palms up. Close your eyes. Your legs should be about eighteen inches apart.

This pose is done between asanas to allow the body to rest completely and experience the benefit of the pose just performed.

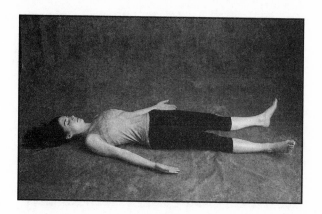

❈ BHUJANGASANA (COBRA POSE) ❈

To prepare, lie on your stomach in *Savasana* (Relaxation Pose), your arms alongside your body and your cheek to one side. Your legs should be about seventeen inches apart. Bring your forehead to the floor. Place your palms on the floor, below your shoulders, elbows raised and close to your body. Relax all your muscles completely. Bring your legs close together with your toes pointed.

Now slowly raise your head and bend your neck back as far as possible. Slowly raise your chest, bending your vertebrae backward one by one. Keep your elbows bent. Inhale while rising, breathe normally in the pose and exhale coming down. Hold for ten seconds. Repeat.

Clinical Benefits

Stimulates the thyroid gland at the base of throat, helping to stabilize metabolism and lower blood cholesterol. The back muscles are strengthened. The spine becomes more supple and the chest expands, promoting oxygen and circulation into the lungs and heart. The cranial nerves at the base of the skull are stimulated, promoting activity and tone. The thymus gland in the center of the chest is stimulated, helping to strengthen the immune function. Backache caused by strain, constipation and flatulence are relieved. Vertebrae displaced in the spine are subtly adjusted. In women, the ovaries and uterus are toned. Various utero-ovarian complaints can be relieved.

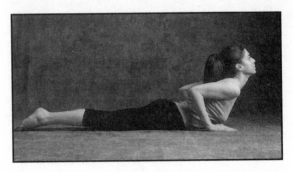

SAVASANA

❀ ARDDHASALABASANA (HALF LOCUST POSE) ❀

Lie facedown with your chin on the floor. Tuck your arms beneath your body, palms up, beneath your thighs. Do not bend your elbows. Keep your toes pointed. Raise your right leg without bending the knee. Allow all your weight to rest on your chest and arms. Slowly lower the leg. Relax. Do the same with the left leg. Turn your head to the side and rest. Keep your arms in place and return your chin to the floor. Repeat. Perform twice with each leg.

Clinical Benefits

The back, pelvis and abdomen are toned and strengthened, helping in the treatment of lower-back weakness, tightness and spasm. The disk space between the spinal vertebrae is stretched, helping to promote spinal alignment. The sympathetic nervous system—the portion of the nervous system devoted to arousal for fight or flight, located in the mid back—is balanced, helping in the treatment of heart disease. Pressure increases in the heart and lungs, helping in their elasticity and lymph drainage. This pose increases circulation and massages the prostate or the uterus and ovaries, helpful in the treatment of prostate or uterine disease.

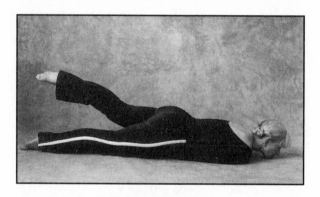

SAVASANA

❁ SALABASANA (LOCUST POSE) ❁

Lie facedown with your chin against the floor. Tuck the arms underneath the body, with the palms up, underneath the thighs. Try to make the elbows touch. Keep the toes pointed. Inhale and retain the breath. Stiffen the body and raise both legs without bending the knees. Allow the entire weight of the body to rest on the chest and arms. Hold the pose for as long as you can comfortably retain the breath. Slowly lower the legs, exhale and relax. Repeat once in the beginning. Hold for ten seconds, or according to capacity.

CAVEAT: More advanced practitioners can begin this pose by clenching the fists underneath the thighs.

Clinical Benefits

Releases tension in the lower back caused by prolonged sitting, which induces stress in the intervertebral disk space and inpedes circulatory activity necessary for maintenance and repair. In addition, this pose applies pressure to the stomach that has been measured at 70–80 mm of mercury, providing massage that is therapeutic for digestion and healthy elimination. The uterus and ovaries in women and the prostate gland in men also benefit by increased circulation. Circulation and lymph drainage is promoted in the heart and lungs. The increased blood flow to the upper body helps improve the facial complexion.

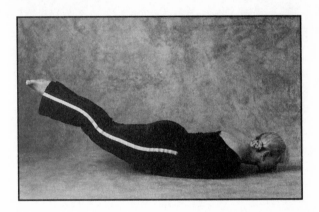

SAVASANA

🌀 DHANYURASANA (BOW POSE) 🌀

Lie facedown with your forehead against the floor. Bring your heels into your buttocks and reach back. Keeping your arms straight, grasp your feet, ankles or lower calves. Gently stretch your heels toward your buttocks, stretching your thigh muscles. Raise your head and chest and, if you can, gently raise your thighs off the floor, allowing the entire weight of your body to fall on your abdomen. Inhale while rising. Breathe normally in the pose. Hold for ten seconds or as long as is comfortable.

To come out of the pose, exhale slowly as you release your legs and slowly lower your chest and head to the floor. Turn your head to the side and relax in Savasana (see page 9) with your arms alongside your body.

To begin with, perform once. As you become more proficient in the pose, do it twice. Because this is a somewhat strenuous pose and requires flexibility in the legs, the beginner should perform it in stages. First, keep your forehead on the floor and just see if you can grasp your ankles or lower calves. If there is a lot of tension or you feel the strain, allow your legs to relax with your heels against your buttocks. This will stretch your thighs and calves. Then, if possible, straighten your arms and gently raise your thighs. After that, if you can, raise your head and chest off the floor. If you need to, gradually work into the pose, little by little each day. As your legs become more flexible, you can begin raising your head and chest. Be patient with yourself.

CAVEAT: Do not pull your legs up by bending your elbows. Keep your arms straight. Those suffering from high blood pressure, hernia or an ulcer in the stomach or intestines should avoid doing this pose.

Clinical Benefits

Stretches the posterior muscles of the lower back and pelvis—primarily the *latissimus dorsi* along the spine and the gluteus muscles in the buttocks. It massages the abdominal organs and digestive tract, improving circulation and helping to prevent and treat constipation. By facilitating circulation to the pancreas, this pose helps stabilize blood sugar levels. The muscles in the chest and upper back are also stretched, increasing blood flow to the lungs and heart.

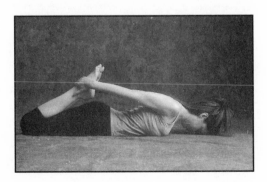
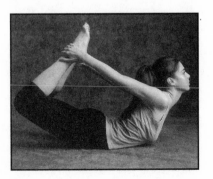

🌀 JANUSIRASANA (HEAD-TO-KNEE POSE) 🌀

Sit on the floor with your legs outstretched. Bring your left heel into the groin area with the sole of your left foot resting against your right inner thigh. Lock your thumbs and raise your arms overhead, stretching your spine up.

Look up at your hands, keep your head aligned between your arms and bend forward over your extended leg. If you can, bring your face to your knee while grasping your extended foot with both hands. Otherwise, bend as far over as your body allows and relax in that position, grasping your shin, calf or knee. Most important, don't strain or force your body forward. As your body relaxes into the pose, you'll find your flexibility level will gradually improve. Keep the leg straight.

Repeat the pose, bending over the left leg. Perform once with each leg. Hold for a maximum of ten seconds.

Clinical Benefits

Helps to relieve constipation. Stimulates the parasympathetic nerves, toning the parasympathetic nervous system and increasing blood flow into the heart, helping in the treatment of heart disease. Reduces plaque in the coronary arteries and lowers cholesterol. Because of the improved circulation and gentle massaging of the lower bowel, the medical benefits of this pose include the prevention and treatment of constipation and hemorrhoids. The additional stimulation to the parasympathetic nervous system also contributes to improved bowel action and relief of constipation.

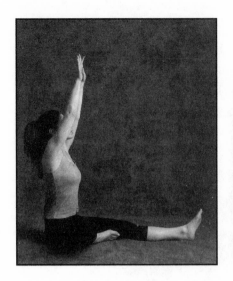
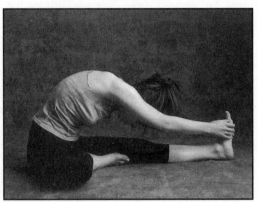

SAVASANA

❀ PASCHIMOTHANASANA (FULL FORWARD BEND) ❀

Lie on your back. Stretch your arms over your head, if you can do so comfortably, and lock your thumbs. Slowly raise your arms, head and chest, sitting up into an upright position. If you find this too difficult, just sit up comfortably, then raise your arms above your head.

Slowly bend forward over your legs as far as you can comfortably go. Grasp your legs wherever you can reach comfortably—your ankles, calves or thighs. Relax your face into your knees if you are able to. Otherwise, relax your head to your chest. Relax in this position, breathing normally, for ten seconds. Do not bend your knees.

When coming out of this pose, lock your thumbs and stretch out over your legs, then rise into an upright position. Bring your hands to your lap and lie back comfortably in a supine position.

Clinical Benefits

Acts in a manner similar to the Head-to-Knee Pose. It stimulates, massages and relaxes the "pelvic bowl." The Full Forward Bend in particular stretches the sacroiliac junction, helpful in the treatment of lower backache as well as sciatica, the painful pinching of the root to the sciatic nerve that can manifest as pain in one or both buttocks or down one or both legs.

CAVEAT: Do not practice this pose if you have a disease of the abdominal viscera or enlargement of the liver or spleen.

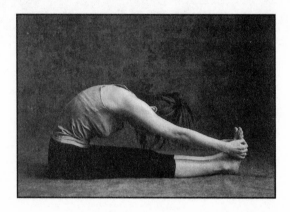

SAVASANA

❀ HALASANA (PLOW POSE) ❀

Lie on your back, keeping your hands alongside the body and palms pressed firmly against the floor. Hold the breath and slowly raise the legs without bending the knees. When the legs are raised to approximately a 90-degree angle, raise the hips and the lower part of the back, bringing the legs to a vertical position to the floor. Then exhale and lower the legs over your head and touch the floor with your toes.

As a variation, bring the knees alongside the head with your arms wrapped behind them.

To come out of the pose, stretch your legs away from your shoulders and head and slowly roll the spine, vertebra by vertebra, to the floor. If necessary, bend your knees as you recline to the floor slowly and easefully.

Clinical Benefits

Effective in releasing tight shoulder muscles as well as the paraspinals of the neck that can become fatigued from holding up the weight of your head. In addition, the Plow Pose stimulates the portion of the parasympathetic nervous system located in the neck, helping to balance it with the sympathetic nervous system. It tones the thyroid gland at the base of the throat and promotes spinal elasticity and spinal nerves, a prerequisite for remaining young. The gentle pressure that is applied to the stomach helps to massage and increase circulation into the digestive system, promoting digestion and healthy bowel function. The liver, spleen and pancreas also receive increased energy and blood flow.

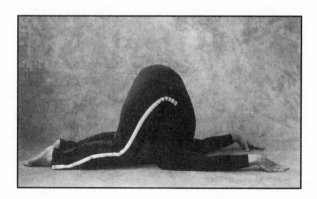

SARVANGASANA (SHOULDERSTAND)
STANDARD VERSION

Adjust your clothing to loosen any restrictions in movement. Lie on your back with your feet together and your arms alongside your body, palms down. Inhale, straighten your legs and lift them over your head in a horizontal position as shown in the illustration. (If necessary, bend your knees in order to raise them over your head.) Then straighten your legs into a vertical position, keeping them together. Bring your palms to your lower back for support. Begin breathing normally. Keep the chin tucked into your chest. Hold for two to three minutes.

To come out of the pose, lower your legs over your head, parallel to the floor. Bring the arms to the floor for support. Slowly roll the spine to the floor, keeping the legs straight if you can. Otherwise, bend the knees as you come down. Continue breathing normally.

The mental focus in this pose is the base of the throat. Do not sneeze, cough, swallow or yawn while in the pose to avoid straining your throat or rupturing small blood vessels.

Clinical Benefits

Stimulates the thyroid gland and stabilizes the metabolism. Increases circulation into all the major glands and organs, including the pituary and pineal glands, the heart, lungs, kidneys, liver and spleen. Increases circulation into and tones the ovaries and uterus in women, helping with feminine disorders. Reduces abdominal fat. Tones the facial nerves and muscles by increasing circulation into them. Balances the active aspect of the nervous system—the sympathetic nervous system—with the relaxing component, the parasympathetic. Parasympathetic nerve fibers are located in the neck and lower back and are stimulated when stretched. Sympathetic fibers, located in the mid back, are often over-activated by stress. This action helps reestablish equilibrium, creating a state of deep relaxation.

CAVEAT: The Shoulderstand, while considered the most beneficial Hatha yoga pose, involves the greatest difficulty level. Be careful to go into and come out of the pose slowly. If you're unable to get into the full pose, modify it by elevating your legs in either a supported or unsupported position (i.e., using a chair or the wall—see page 104). No matter which variation your body is able to do, you're gaining the benefit of reversing the pull of gravity on your system and increasing the flow of blood and vital energy to all your organs and glands.

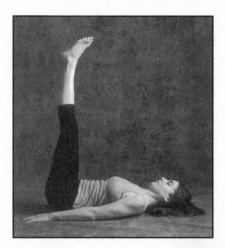

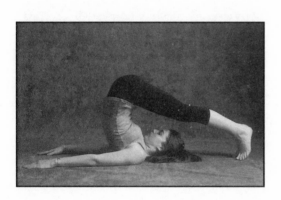

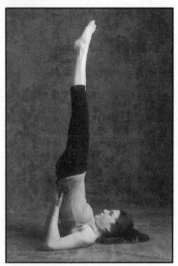

SARVANGASANA (SHOULDERSTAND)
MODIFIED VERSION

(a) Lie on your back with your legs elevated on a chair. Hold this position for three minutes, or come out of the pose sooner if you become uncomfortable.

(b) Lie on your back with your legs elevated on a wall.

Use these modifications if you have severe high blood pressure, back pain, neck or shoulder injuries or other physiological limitations. Postoperative patients should use either of these modifications for two months before attempting to do the standard version.

SAVASANA

❀ MATSYASANA (FISH POSE) ❀

Lie flat on the floor with your palms pressed against the sides of your thighs. Shift your bodyweight to your elbows and raise your head and trunk. Arch your chest and lower the crown of your head to the floor, creating a "bridge" between your buttocks and head. Expand your chest as much as possible and bring a smile to your lips to break up tension in your jaw.

To come out of the pose, place your bodyweight on your elbows again and raise your head gently. Then slowly roll your spine to the floor. Deep breathing through your nose enhances the benefit of the practice. Do not retain the breath. Hold for approximately ten seconds.

CAVEAT: Do not swallow while doing this pose, as it may cause you to gag or experience a choking sensation. If you feel like coughing or sneezing, come out of the pose before doing so. Do not do this posture if you have a headache or fever.

Clinical Benefits
Increases circulation to the lungs and heart. By extending the cervical and thoracic spine backward, the muscles of the neck, upper back and chest are stretched and stimulated, increasing flexibility and circulation. Because it improves circulation to the thyroid, the Fish Pose helps this gland regulate itself, keeping it from becoming either over- or underactive, thereby stabilizing the metabolism.

As reported in the *Journal of the American Medical Association,* the Fish Pose has been clinically recognized to be effective in the treatment of asthma and bronchial conditions.

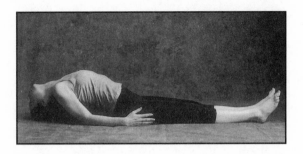

SAVASANA

PAVANAMUKTASANA (WIND ELIMINATION)

Lie flat on your back. Raise both legs to your chest while drawing in a deep breath through your nose. Hold the breath. Raise your head and bring it to your knees. Exhale slowly, release your legs and lie back on the floor with your arms and legs extended.

Clinical Benefits
Relieves strain and tightness in the lower back. It massages the abdominal organs and digestive tract, pushing the contents of the bowel along. In this way, any accumulated gas is expelled, relieving the pressure of flatulence.

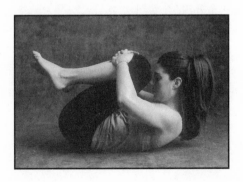

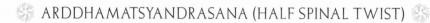 ARDDHAMATSYANDRASANA (HALF SPINAL TWIST)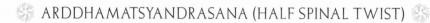

Sit on the floor and bring your knees to your chest. Extend your right leg straight up. Cross your right foot over your left knee, placing the sole of your right foot flat on the floor. Sitting up straight, bring your right knee close to your chest. Now extend your arms in front of you, locking your thumbs and twisting to the right. Unlock your thumbs and place your right hand on the floor behind you, close to your body, with your fingers pointing away from you. Place your left arm between your trunk and your right knee (i.e., on the outside of your right knee) and press your knee to the right. You can also wrap your left arm around your right knee, bringing it close to your chest. Slowly twist your head and trunk to the right and look over your right shoulder. Hold for ten seconds.

Slowly unwind, coming back to center. Bring both knees to your chest, then repeat the pose with your left leg.

Clinical Benefits

Increases circulation into the liver, spleen, kidneys, gallbladder and adrenal glands. By increasing pressure and circulation to the abdominal cavity and organs through the twisting motion, it helps to relieve constipation. It tones the sympathetic nerves and ganglia (nerve bundles) in the mid and lower back, thereby reducing stress levels and helping in the treatment of obesity. It also strengthens the deep (lower) and superficial (upper and middle) muscles of the back, which hold up the spine and keep the vertebrae in place.

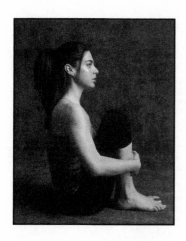 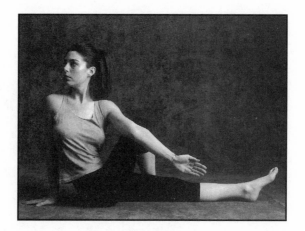

SAVASANA

🏵 YOGA MUDRA (YOGIC SEAL) 🏵

Sit on the floor in a comfortable cross-legged position. Place your hands behind your back and grasp your right wrist with the left hand. Inhale, slowly bend forward and touch the floor with your forehead first and then, gradually, your chin. If you have only a limited range of motion, just relax forward as far as you can and relax your chin to your chest. The focus is the center of your forehead. On the exhalation, stretch your chin out and slowly rise.

Clinical Benefits

By gently massaging the digestive tract, this pose aids in moving food along, helping prevent constipation. By increasing circulation to the pancreas, it helps improve this gland's function, thus assisting in the prevention and treatment of obesity. The sympathetic nerves—the portion of the nervous system located in the mid back, consisting of nerve fibers and ganglia (masses of nerve cell bodies located along the spinal column)—are stimulated, as well as the parasympathetic nerves in the lower back. This activity helps relax the body and center the mind. It also strengthens both the deep *erector spinae* muscles that support the lumbar spine and the superficial—*latissimus dorsi*—muscles of the mid back.

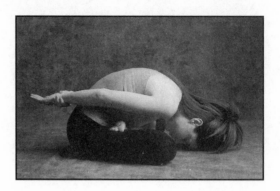

❀ YOGA NIDRA (DEEP RELAXATION) ❀

Lie on your back in a comfortable supine position with your arms and legs extended. Your legs should be about a foot and a half apart, and your arms a few inches away from the body. Close your eyes and, breathing through your nose, begin relaxing into your position. Bring your awareness to your right leg and foot. Tense the leg. Lift it off the floor a few inches. Tense a little tighter and let it drop. Roll it from side to side and just forget about it. Repeat with the left leg.

Now inhale and tense your pelvis and buttocks. Squeeze the tension out. Most of us hold a lot of stress in this area, which can lead to disorders in the reproductive system as well as in the pelvis and hips. Now inhale and fill your stomach with air. Hold it for a few moments and then release through your mouth. Just let it gush out. Inhale again, filling your stomach with air. Then bring it into your chest. Hold it. Open your mouth and let it gush out. Experience the warm sensation of the release.

Bring your awareness to your right hand and arm. Inhale, close your hand into a gentle fist and begin tensing tightly all the way to your shoulder. Then release. Repeat with your left hand and arm.

Inhale and raise your shoulders to your ears. Hold for a moment. Then release. Turn your head from side to side slowly. Then center and relax. Bring your awareness to your face. Open your mouth and drop your jaw. Move it from side to side. Then center and relax. Now tense your face into a tight "prune" face. And release. Open your mouth wide and extend your tongue as far as you can. And then relax. Your body should be completely relaxed and free of tension at this point.

To begin the second phase of the practice, without moving, bring your mental awareness to your feet. Begin mentally relaxing your feet. Now bring your mental awareness up your entire body, relaxing each part until you reach your head. Once your body is free of all stress, bring your mental awareness to your breath. Begin observing the flow of your breath. Just watch the gentle inhalation and exhalation. You'll notice that your breath becomes increasingly subtle. It might seem like you're not breathing at all. Don't worry. You are.

Just watch yourself becoming more and more relaxed as your breath becomes more "invisible" and subtle. I have known some clients to become afraid at this point, when the breath is very still. It's not an uncommon reaction. If you can, just keep relaxing through it. The breath is just deepening. You are breathing on a subtler level that is much more therapeutic than the breathing we're accustomed to.

At this point, when your breath is quite still, bring your awareness to your mind. Begin watching your mind. Begin watching your thoughts as they enter and leave your mind. You most likely will find that your mind begins to fill with thoughts at this point, particularly if you are new to this practice. It's a common experience. The important thing is not to push the thoughts away. Don't force anything. Just continue watching the phenomenon as though you're watching a film. After doing this practice a few times you will find that eventually your mind will begin to relax and let go. Then you'll begin to experience a very relaxed, blissful quality within yourself that you will find will help to rejuvenate and restore your energy. This is where the healing takes place—in this very subtle and peaceful energy within you.

In a formal class, for optimal benefit it's customary for the silent relaxation part of the practice to last for ten to fifteen minutes. When doing it on your own you can customize the time to accommodate your schedule.

There is an audiotape of the Yoga Nidra practice recorded by Swami Satchidananda that I use with my cardiac patients at Cedars-Sinai Medical Center and many of my private clients (see Resources for details).

As you come out of your relaxation, slowly bring your awareness back to your breath and let it gradually deepen. Imagine that you're breathing all the way into your feet. Let your awareness rise through your body, waking up all the parts until you reach your head. Then begin gently moving all parts of your body. Observe their relaxed and eased quality.

Now rise slowly and begin preparation for the pranayama (breathing practices).

Clinical Benefits
Reduces stress in the muscles, organs and nervous system. Stabilizes the parasympathetic nervous system. By stabilizing the parasympathetic nervous system and lowering blood pressure, in particular, this practice is highly recommended for treatment of cardiovascular disease because it allows the heart to rest more deeply. By reducing stress levels, it is also known to strengthen the immune system.

Further exposition on the benefits and technique of yoga nidra is included in the section on meditation in Part II (pages 206–208).

Pranayama (Breathing Practices)

Pranayama means control of prana, our life force, the vital energy that is present everywhere and that produces the most subtle movements in our mental and physical systems and in nature. As my guru has explained, by the regular practice of yoga we are not only able to control and direct the prana that functions within us, we're able to direct and control the universal prana as well. This is done through our thought—the agent that directs the prana.

The breath is the external manifestation of prana. We breathe about fifteen times a minute. In a normal breath, we take in and give out approximately 1 pint of air. By applying the yoga pranayama techniques, we begin to optimize this intake by adding a little extra effort to inhale further. More of the small grapelike sacks of the lungs, the alveoli, are opened up, so the body can expel increased amounts of carbon dioxide and take in more oxygen. You end up feeling more refreshed.

Since oxygen is vital in supporting the cardiovascular system, the neuroendocrine system, the immune system and the metabolic system, pranayama practices are critical because they maximize our intake of air, thus strengthening and enhancing these systems and preventing and treating diseases related to them.

To understand the difference between normal oxygen intake and that maximized by pranayama practice, we can use the results of clinical measurements. If you were to measure a normal intake of air in cubic centimeters (cc), we usually exchange about 500 cc with each breath After as little as six weeks of regular practice of the pranayama techniques, clinical studies have shown that the average breath increases to approximately 700 cc. This increase in capacity significantly promotes vitality and overall health.

All of these breathing techniques help to balance the sympathetic and parasympathetic nervous systems, stabilizing heart rate and blood pressure. They produce a profound calming effect on the mind and body and decrease sympathetic nervous system stimulation. They also balance the availability of energy to your system.

DEERGA SWASAM (DEEP BREATHING)

Sit in a comfortable cross-legged position with your eyes gently closed. Exhale completely through your nose. Place your right hand on your chest and your left hand on your abdomen. Inhale and fill your abdominal area with air. As you do this, your left

hand will begin to rise but your right hand will not. After filling your abdomen with air, keep inhaling and allow more air to fill your lower chest. This will cause your right hand to rise. Your rib cage will expand as you inhale. Continue inhaling, bringing the air higher into your chest to your collarbone, causing it to rise.

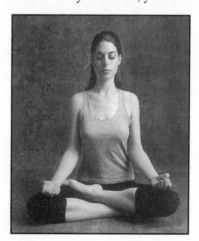

On the exhalation, slowly expel the air, deflating your upper chest, rib cage and abdomen. Bring your abdomen toward your spine. Do this for at least one minute.

KAPALA BATHI (SKULL SHINING)

Exhale completely through your nose. Inhale and produce a quick contraction of your abdomen, expelling the air. Then inhale and expel the air again. Repeat rapidly seven or eight times. The inhalation and exhalation should have equal force. Have a long exhalation. Rest for a moment and begin a second round. Repeat three times. As you continue your practice, increase your capacity.

Clinical Benefits

Kapala Bathi brings heat to the body when it's cold. It improves digestion, removes phlegm and helps in the prevention and treatment of asthma and other respiratory diseases. It exhilarates blood circulation and energizes the entire body quickly. It can also help in the treatment of depression.

NADDI SUDDHI (ALTERNATE NOSTRIL BREATHING): STAGE ONE

Sit in a comfortable cross-legged position. Make a loose fist with your right hand. Release your thumb and last two fingers. Relax your right arm against your chest and close your right nostril with your right thumb. Slowly exhale as much air as possible without strain through your left nostril. Then inhale through your left nostril and close it with the last two fingers of your right hand. Exhale through your right nostril.

Upon inhalation, be sure to expand your stomach to full capacity to allow as much air as possible to enter your lungs. Upon exhalation, completely empty your lungs. Alternate your breathing this way a few times for as long as is comfortable. Then have a final exhalation through your right nostril and let your breath return to normal. Sit for a moment and observe the peaceful and calming effect of this practice on your system.

Clinical Benefits

Reduces stress from the sympathetic nervous system and balances it with the parasympathetic nervous system, allowing the heart to rest deeply. Helps to stabilize the sinus rhythm of the heart and to alleviate depression and anxiety and strengthens memory.

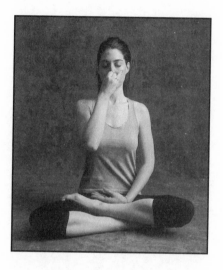

CHIN MUDRA (SYMBOL OF WISDOM)

Rest the hands on the corresponding knees. Stretch out the upturned palms. On each hand touch the tip of the thumb with the tip of the index finger. Point the remaining three fingers on each hand downward.

NOTE: In this position, all the fingers represent something. The thumb represents the universal, or higher self. The index finger represents the individual self. The middle finger represents the ego. The ring finger represents the illusion of the mind. The fourth, or little, finger represents all the worldly actions and their reactions.

During Chin Mudra, all of the individual self symbolically renounces all worldliness and rises toward the higher self. While watching the actions of the individual self, the higher self gracefully bends down to meet it, thus forming the symbolic union of the universal and individual selves. It is helpful during meditation to sit in this position during your spiritual practice as a reminder of the purpose of life. Gradually the awareness and connection with the universal or "spiritual" self will begin to integrate into your daily life, helping to inform all of your actions and relationships.

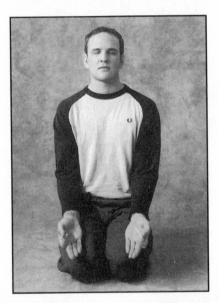

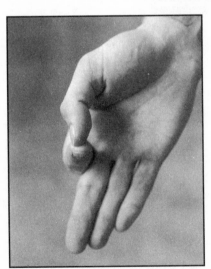

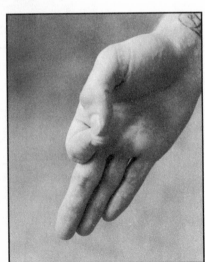

Specific Poses to Protect Your Body from Disease

Every human being is the author of his own health or disease.
—Sri Swami Sivananda

Our bodies are our gardens—our wills are our gardeners.
—William Shakespeare

ow we will take a closer look at how yoga helps protect the entire body from potential health problems. For each system of the body discussed in this section, specific poses (*asanas*) and deep relaxation (*yoga nidra*) and breathing techniques (*pranayama*) are described that have been shown to help prevent the onset of diseases and symptoms that can negatively affect that system. As stated in the introduction, yoga is a complete science; the postures, or asanas, interact to create a synergy of healing for the entire body. No one or two postures isolated from the entire set will "heal" or restore a particular bodily system or organ. No organ is an island. They work together synergistically to create, ideally, total health.

In the Eastern tradition of medicine, the approach to health, like the science of yoga, is holistic. It is understood that the body's intricate system of organs, muscles, nerves and glands is synergistic—i.e., the lungs support the heart, the kidneys support the lungs, the heart supports the colon and the digestive system, and so on. The systems are interrelated and interact with one another to achieve maximum function and health. Additionally, as you will see, the mind and the breath are inextricably connected to the body in sustaining both mental and physical health and well-being. Therefore, the asanas described in this section should be done only as a supplemental adjunct to the thirty-minute Yoga for Health Practice Set I (see pages 3–30). While these designated asanas, strategic for particular systems, will provide an added strength to each system, in order to achieve the maximum benefit of optimal health all of the asanas included in the complete Yoga for Health program should be done at least once, and preferably three times, a week.

> *If the mind, that rules the body, ever so far forgets itself as to trample on its slave, the slave is never generous enough to forgive the injury, but will rise and smite the oppressor.*
>
> —HENRY WADSWORTH LONGFELLOW

NOTE: As described in the thirty-minute Yoga for Health Practice Set, *Savasana* (Relaxation Pose)—in which you lie on your back or stomach, legs extended and about seventeen inches apart—should be done between asanas to allow your body to rest completely and experience the benefit of the pose just performed.

Conclude each of the following dedicated sessions with a short pranayama practice as described in the thirty-minute Yoga for Health Practice Set I (pages 3–30) to allow your body to relax further and support the effects of the asana program you've done.

The Cardiovascular and Circulatory Systems

PRIMARY ORGAN: *Heart*

Related disease conditions
Coronary artery disease
High blood pressure
Hypertension/Stress

Cardiomyopathy

Atrial fibrillation

Varicose veins

Angina

Atherosclerosis

Congestive heart failure

Shock

The Role of Stress

Both Dr. Ornish's Heart Disease Reversal Program and the Cedars-Sinai Medical Center Preventive and Rehabilitative Center place great emphasis on using yoga to help reduce stress leading to heart disease. Patients do the full format of techniques for an hour each day.

Stress can cause the arteries of the heart to constrict and precipitate a heart attack, even in young people who do not have a buildup of cholesterol or plaque. Stress has a way of sneaking up on us and can take subtle forms in our lives. In many cases the symptoms are masked until it's too late. The following story about one of my patients at Cedars-Sinai Medical Center is typical of how yoga can dramatically impact rehabilitation from a life-threatening acute condition.

A successful film producer was at the height of his career when he went to see his physician for a routine exam and found out he had five blocked arteries requiring quadruple bypass surgery. He had had no idea that his health was in so perilous a state. He was physically active. He played tennis and was a regular on the Aspen slopes. He wasn't short of breath and did not experience chest pain. But he had recently lost a good friend to heart disease, and in his working life was producing five films. He wasn't doing any

The practice of Hatha Yoga builds up strength within the system. You tone the muscles, organs, endocrine glands, spine and all the nerve centers. Unlike many exercises the asanas do not cause strain. They are done very gently, with grace and ease.

—SRI SWAMI SATCHIDANANDA

kind of stress management. At the time he considered yoga, meditation and anything related "New Age woo-wooism." After his surgery he started on an aggressive course of yoga therapy with me and modified his diet according to the recommendations of Cedars-Sinai cardiologist Dr. C. Noel Bairey Merz. Within three months he was back at work and had resumed the flow of his life . . . but with a new perspective. And a radically different perspective on yoga!

Prana is the vital energy or force that causes movement. All movement everywhere—even the movement within the atom, even the movement of thought—is caused by prana, the cosmic energy. The practice of pranayama leads to the control, regulation and mastery of this vital force.

—SRI SWAMI SATCHIDANANDA

Harvard Medical School has produced a profile of stresses found to precede dangerous arrhythmias. Dr. Thomas Graboys relates that "a complex interplay of the sympathetic-parasympathetic axis may affect sympathetic neural traffic to the heart and change the threshold of ventricular fibrillation." In other words, the interaction of the sympathetic (alertness) and parasympathetic (relaxation) portions of our nervous systems may affect the ability of the heart to beat regularly. Dangerous patterns may lead to a heart attack. Dr. Ornish notes that heart attacks, congestive heart failure and angina have all been found to be adversely affected by emotional factors. For example, in his book *Love and Survival*, he relates that the degree of love and intimacy in our lives is inversely proportional to heart disease rates. People who live alone have double the risk of having a heart attack. Joining a group yoga class may reduce this risk. Dr. Ornish discusses the relationship of this dynamic in depth in his books *Stress, Diet and Your Heart* and *Dr. Dean Ornish's Program for Reversing Heart Disease*.

However, not everyone can attend a group class or feels comfortable in one. I have many private patients who do not. As Swami Satchidananda reminds us in his teachings, just by doing a regular practice of yoga we begin to realize that we are never really alone. And in his book *To Know Your Self*, Swami Satchidananda gives a practical explanation of how, by doing yoga and meditating, you begin to unite with the universal love and peace within yourself, which he refers to as the "inside comfortor." It frees you from the bonds of attachment and allows you to experience the wealth of inner peace and health.

The following specific asanas are noted by medical experts to be directly related to strengthening the cardiovascular system and preventing heart and circulation-related disease.

Recommended Asanas

❧ BHUJANGASANA (COBRA POSE) ❧

Applies pressure on the lungs and heart, encouraging an increase in lymph flow, which may help protect against heart disease.

Some medical authorities feel that the flow of lymph may help determine how much plaque builds up in the coronary arteries.

To begin, lie on your back and relax in Savasana (Relaxation Pose) for a few moments. Then turn over into Savasana on your stomach with your arms alongside your body and your cheek to one side. Your legs should be about seventeen inches apart. Bring your forehead to the floor. Place your palms on the floor, below your shoulders, elbows raised and close to your body. Relax all your muscles completely. Bring your legs close together with your toes pointed.

Now slowly raise your head and bend your neck back as far as possible. Slowly raise your chest, bending your vertebrae backward one by one. Keep your elbows bent. Inhale while raising up, breathe normally in the pose and exhale coming down. Hold for ten seconds. Repeat.

I am a firm believer that all uneasiness (dis-ease) in the body results from a variety of causes: stress, improper diet, etc.—thereby creating toxins in the body and decreasing proper oxidation for the cells. This is a precursor to all disease. Yoga can be to the body what love is to life. Additionally, no one should ever be in pain in a yoga class. If they are, they have the wrong teacher. Yoga has had a significant impact on my life and continues to play an important role not only in my physical and mental well-being but in enhancing my spiritual destiny as well.

—DIANE LADD, ACTRESS

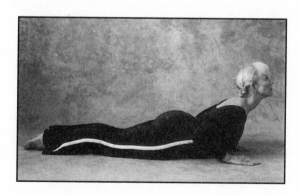

🕉 JANUSIRASANA (HEAD-TO-KNEE POSE) 🕉

Sit on the floor with your legs outstretched. Bring your left heel into the groin area with the sole of your left foot resting against your right inner thigh. Lock your thumbs and raise your arms overhead, stretching your spine up.

> *A light heart lives long.*
>
> —WILLIAM SHAKESPEARE

Look up at your hands, keep your head aligned between your arms and bend forward over your extended leg. Bring your face to your knee, keeping your leg straight. Relax into the pose. Avoid straining. Repeat the pose, bending over your left leg. Perform once with each leg. Hold for a maximum of ten seconds.

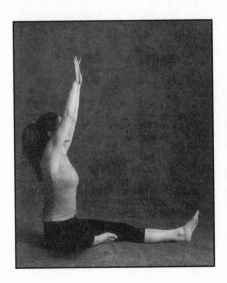
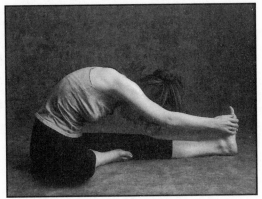

🕉 SARVANGASANA (SHOULDERSTAND) 🕉

With regard to the change in the body's physiology with this pose, for the first thirty seconds or so the heart rate increases. However, within about a minute it decreases, producing a feeling of relaxation and calm. Resting your chin on your chest stimulates the pressure-sensitive "baroceptor" cells located in the lining of the arteries of your neck. When stimulated, they send a signal to the brain to lower blood pressure and pulse, thereby relieving tension in the cardiovascular system by allowing the heart and arteries to rest more deeply.

Varicose veins and hemorrhoids result when the constant pressure of gravity exceeds what the valves in the veins can handle. A daily Shoulderstand may act as a preventive technique for these and other circulatory-related conditions.

> *Nature does require her time of preservation, which perforce I her frail son amongst my brethren mortal must give my attendance to.*
>
> —WILLIAM SHAKESPEARE

Loosen your clothing to avoid any restrictions in movement. Lie on your back with your feet together and your arms alongside your body, palms down. Inhale, straighten your legs and lift them over your head in a horizontal position as shown in the illustration. (If necessary, bend your knees in order to raise them over your head.) Straighten your legs into a vertical position, keeping them together. Bring your palms to your lower back for support. Breathe normally. Keep your chin tucked into your chest. Hold for two to three minutes.

To come out of this pose, lower your legs over your head, parallel to the floor. Bring your arms to the floor for support. Slowly roll your spine to the floor, keeping your legs straight if you can. Otherwise, bend your knees as you come down. Continue breathing normally.

> *Stress is your body's way of saying you haven't worked enough unpaid overtime.*
>
> —SCOTT ADAMS, *DILBERT*

Remember, if this is too difficult or challenging, you can gain the same benefits from doing the modified version of the Shoulderstand described on page 103.

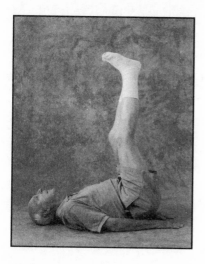
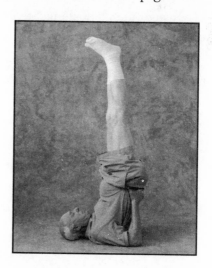

❀ MATSYASANA (FISH POSE) ❀

The Fish Pose is a complementary pose to the Shoulderstand, and in his classic *Integral Yoga Hatha* manual, Sri Swami Satchidananda recommends that this pose be done right after you do the Shoulderstand.

The Fish Pose stretches the thyroid, neck and shoulder muscles in the opposite direction to the Shoulderstand. This opposite stretching is important because the muscles are massaged in a continuing circulation pattern, helping prevent congestion. These areas can then obtain optimum nutrition and conduct more efficient maintenance and repair. Again, it balances the parasympathetic and sympathetic nervous systems. Because it shortens the space between the posterior aspects of the vertebrae in the neck, it should be done very slowly. Try to stretch your neck out as you stretch it back.

The best comforter is inside us. If we feel that Presence in us, where is the need for any other comfort? All other kinds of comfort are temporary. They come, and there will be a time when they must go. Don't depend on something that comes from the outside. Outside things are never going to make you happy. And it should be that way, so that one day you will realize that there is always someone to love and comfort us inside.

—Sri Swami Satchidananda

Lie flat on the floor with your palms pressed against the sides of your thighs. Shift your bodyweight to your elbows and raise your head and trunk. Arch your chest and lower the crown of your head to the floor, creating a "bridge" between your buttocks and head. Expand your chest as much as possible and bring a smile to your lips to break up tension in your jaw.

To come out of the pose, place your bodyweight on your elbows again and raise your head gently. Then slowly roll your spine to the floor. Deep breathing through your nose enhances the benefit of the practice. Do not retain the breath. Hold for approximately ten seconds.

CAVEAT: Do not swallow while doing this pose as it might cause you to choke. If you feel like coughing or sneezing, come out of the pose before doing so. Do not do this posture if you have a headache or fever.

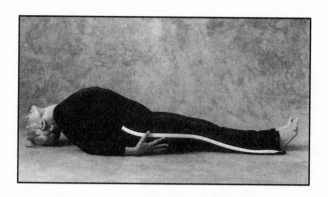

Yoga Nidra (Deep Relaxation)

Deep relaxation alone has been used to treat many diseases and is recommended as part of any preventive and therapeutic health program. Because much of its emphasis is on reducing stress, deep relaxation is considered by physicians such as Dr. McLanahan and Dr. Ornish to be a key in strengthening and supporting the cardiovascular system.

The guided relaxation has been demonstrated to affect both biochemical and nervous discharge in the direction of a more relaxed state. Blood pressure falls and breathing slows. The process is physiologically more restful than a good night's sleep, yet takes only a few minutes.

Consider how much more you often suffer from your anger and grief, than from those very things for which you are angry and grieved.

—Marcus Aurelius Antoninus

In a study by Dr. Chandra Patel in London, patients were guided in a half-hour deep relaxation session three times a week. A control group spent half an hour just lying on a sofa. The experimental group showed a marked drop in blood pressure, and this lowered pressure lasted for a year afterward. The control group showed a small drop in blood pressure, indicating the importance of rest alone as a healing agent.

Lie on your back in a comfortable supine position with your arms and legs extended. Your legs should be about a foot and a half apart, and your arms a few inches away from the body with your palms up. Close your eyes and, breathing through your nose, begin relaxing into your position.

Bring your awareness to your right leg and foot. Tense the leg. Lift it off the floor a few inches. Tense a little tighter and let it drop. Roll it from side to side and just forget about it. Repeat with the left leg.

Now inhale and tense your pelvis and buttocks. Squeeze the tension out. Most of us hold a lot of stress in this area, which can lead to disorders in the reproductive system as well as in the pelvis and hips. Now inhale and fill your stomach with air. Hold it for a few moments and then release through your mouth. Just let it gush out. Inhale again, filling your stomach with air. Then bring it into your chest. Hold it. Open your mouth and let it gush out. Experience the warm sensation of the release. Bring your awareness to your right hand and arm. Inhale, close your hand into a gentle fist and begin tensing tightly all the way to your shoulder. Then release. Repeat with your left hand and arm.

Inhale and raise your shoulders to your ears. Hold for a moment. Then release. Turn your head from side to side slowly. Then center and relax. Bring your awareness to your face. Open your mouth and drop your jaw. Move it from side to side. Then center and relax. Now tense your face into a tight "prune" face. And release. Open your mouth wide and extend your tongue as far as you can. And then relax. Your body should be completely relaxed and free of tension at this point.

To begin the second phase of the practice, without moving, bring your mental awareness to your feet. Begin mentally relaxing your feet. Now bring your mental awareness up your entire body, relaxing each part until you reach your head. Once your body is free of all stress, bring your mental awareness to your breath. Begin observing the flow of your breath. Just watch the gentle inhalation and exhalation.

As you come out of your relaxation, slowly bring your awareness back to your breath and let it gradually deepen. Imagine that you're breathing all the way into your feet. Let your awareness rise through your body, waking up all the parts until

I used to go nuts with rage in my car when somebody would cut me off or perform any of the rude acts we all encounter when driving. I used to chase after guys to yell at them out the window or honk my horn and give them the dirtiest look. Road Rage. No More. When I run into that kind of situation nowadays, some sort of emotional switch automatically turns on and I see an image of my yoga therapist, Nirmala Heriza, leading our yoga group. I mentally go into my three preparatory "oms" and let the monster race away in his BMW. A happier way to go . . . and much, much safer.

—HAL COOPER, EIGHTY, EMMY AWARD–WINNING TV DIRECTOR OF *THAT GIRL*, *ALL IN THE FAMILY* AND *MAUDE*

you reach your head. Then begin gently moving all parts of your body. Observe their relaxed and eased quality.

Now rise slowly and begin preparation for the pranayama.

Pranayama: Breathing Techniques

Breathing is one of the most effective tools in reducing stress. By simply taking a deep breath you can become more relaxed. Breathing can diffuse the most heated emotional situations. I have experienced this many times myself. One day, while researching this book, I received a call from a business associate who was in a very angry mood. No matter what I said, she began yelling at me. As her voice grew louder, my system began to react. My heart raced and my body began to tense. I went into the typical "fight or flight" mode. Rather than try to fight back or hang up mid-sentence (i.e., fight or flee), I began doing some deep breathing. That was all. Just breathing deeply and slowly. The effect was that it kept my mind and nervous system calm and unaffected. Even though I wasn't able to reason with her during the conversation (or even have an opportunity to speak at all!), afterward I wasn't anywhere near as rattled as I would have been had I engaged in an argument. When she called back later, my calm demeanor immediately put her at ease and she was able to continue our conversation in a more reasonable state of mind.

> *Reality is nothing but a collective hunch.*
>
> —LILY TOMLIN

So, besides serving the very basic functions of bringing oxygen to the blood and cells, sustaining the life force and enhancing energy levels, breathing is a tactical tool for preventing high blood pressure, cardiac disease or stroke—conditions that are clinically noted to be caused by emotional stressors such as anger and fear.

Usually we breathe in and out about 500 cubic centimeters of air. After just six weeks of yoga training, the average breath has been recorded at 700 cubic centimeters. This kind of breathing keeps you continuously relaxed.

🟐 DEERGA SWASAM (DEEP BREATHING) 🟐

Exhale completely through your nose. Place your right hand on your chest and your left hand on your abdomen. Inhale and fill your abdominal area with air. As you do this, your left hand will begin to rise but your right hand will not. After filling your abdomen with air, keep inhaling and allow more air to fill your lower chest. This will cause your right hand to rise. Your rib cage will expand as you inhale. Continue inhaling, bringing the air higher into your chest to your collarbone, causing it to rise.

On the exhalation, slowly expel the air, deflating your upper chest, rib cage and abdomen. Bring your abdomen toward the spine. Do this for at least one minute.

🟐 KAPALA BATHI (SKULL SHINING) 🟐

Kabala Bathi is an invigorating practice you can do without exerting much physical energy. The only muscles doing the work are the abdominals (and those in the spine if you're sitting in an unsupported position).

Exhale completely through your nose. Inhale and produce a quick contraction of your abdomen, expelling the air. Then inhale and expel the air again. Repeat the rapid expulsion of air seven or eight times. The inhalation and exhalation should have equal force. Have a long exhalation. Rest for a moment and begin a second round of the practice. Do this three times. As you continue your practice, increase the number of contractions to as many as you feel comfortable with. Be careful not to strain.

🌸 NADDI SUDDHI (NERVE PURIFICATION) 🌸

EEG measurements of subjects performing this exercise demonstrate that it balances activity in the two hemispheres of the brain, which produces an increased sense of relaxation.

Sit in a comfortable cross-legged position. Make a loose fist with your right hand. Release your thumb and last two fingers. Relax your right arm against your chest and close your right nostril with your right thumb. Slowly exhale as much air as possible without strain through your left nostril. Then inhale through your left nostril and close it with the last two fingers of your right hand. Exhale through your right nostril.

Upon inhalation, be sure to expand your stomach to full capacity to allow as much air as possible to enter your lungs. Upon exhalation, completely empty your lungs. Alternate your breathing this way a few times for as long as is comfortable. Then have a final exhalation through your right nostril and let your breath return to normal. Sit for a moment and observe the peaceful and calming effect of this practice on your system.

The Nervous System

CENTRAL NERVOUS SYSTEM

Brain
Spinal cord

Autonomic Nervous System
Relates to the function of the internal organs

The nervous system is made up of the sympathetic nervous system, the parasympathetic nervous system, the autonomic nervous system, the somatic nervous system, and the central nervous system. The sympathetic system controls activity and stress. It emerges from the mid back, and its activity causes the "fight or flight" response. The parasympathetic nervous system is located in the neck and lower back and produces a relaxation response. It reacts in a complementary way to the sympathetic nervous system.

The health of every tissue in the body depends on this system because nerves from the brain and spine go to all the organs and glands of the body. A healthy spine plays a vital role in vitality and rejuvenation.

While the full set of Hatha yoga postures is recommended to increase the health of all these systems, the following postures, relaxation method and breathing techniques can be used in isolation to rebalance, strengthen and tone them.

> *Tension is who you think you should be; relaxation is who you are.*
>
> —CHINESE PROVERB

The somatic nervous system contains both afferent (incoming) and efferent (outgoing) nerves. It receives and processes information passed to it by receptors in the skin, voluntary muscles, tendons, joints, eyes, tongue, nose and ears, giving us the sensations of touch, pain, heat, cold, balance, sight, taste, smell and sound. It allows us to move our arms and legs.

Disease conditions commonly related to the
autonomic and somatic nervous systems

Shingles

Migraines

Substance abuse

Insomnia

ADD (Attention Deficit Disorder)

Anxiety disorders

Fibromyalgia (Chronic Fatigue)

Parkinson's disease

Meningitis

Alzheimer's disease

Epilepsy

Encephalitis

Memory loss

Stroke

Schizophrenia

The proven benefits of yoga have led to its inclusion as an integral component in the medical management of numerous disorders. Preliminary findings indicate that yoga may be used effectively to reduce stress and seizures in patients with epilepsy. For example, Dr. Steven Pacia, M.D., assistant professor of neurology at NYU School of Medicine, is currently conducting a clinical yoga study to evaluate whether yoga can reduce the number of seizures in people with epilepsy and improve their emotional well-being. Dr. Pacia relates that the NYU Comprehensive Epilepsy Center is one of many hospitals around the country offering yoga to their patients. Instructors tailor classes to the abilities of each patient, and even patients who have never exercised enjoy yoga. The classes are structured so that the last half hour is devoted to breathing exercises and meditation. While studies are still in progress, Dr. Pacia and program coordinator Tricia Spoto have received positive feedback from nearly all participants. One of Dr. Pacia's students, an elderly gentleman called Joe, said the following about his experience with the program:

"I began taking part in the Yoga Research Project at NYU Epilepsy Center about two and a half years ago. At that time, I was experiencing two or three seizures over a six-month period, even though I was taking medication [Dilantin, 400 mg per day]. I didn't notice much difference at first, except for an increasing awareness of different parts of my body—those parts we take for granted because we don't use them much. And I became aware of muscular tensions that were caused by my emotional anxieties. The practice helped me identify and release tensions that in the past would build up until they were released by a seizure. I had one seizure about two months after beginning the practice, and then went for nearly a year until one was triggered by my reaction to a personal family difficulty. I have now gone eight months without having a seizure.

> *Perfect health means no weakness anywhere, that is no weakness in the body, or in the mind, or in the relationship between the body and the mind.*
>
> —MAHARISHI MAHESH YOGI

"Because of the epileptic seizures, I had finally given up trying to work as an actor. The 'behind-the-scenes' pressures and anxieties involved were just too much for me; or rather, I allowed them to become too much because I had no tool to control them. That is what yoga has become for me. Now I am singing, which was my first love, and trying to put a cabaret act together. Should the opportunity come, I would definitely try acting again. I take yoga instruction twice a week at NYU Medical Center and practice forty-five minutes to an hour at home on other days. As my instructor has confirmed, I believe that doing it on a daily basis is more beneficial. You actually receive from it what you put into it. It's like buying *The New York Times*—you must read it to be informed. Just buying it isn't enough."

Recommended Asanas

 JANUSIRASANA (HEAD-TO-KNEE POSE)

Massages the parasympathetic nervous system (nerves situated in the lower spine), producing a relaxation effect helpful in the management of anxiety and stress. In addition, the superficial and deep muscles along our spines work very long days to keep the vertebrae upright and in line. This pose helps these muscles relax so they can receive improved circulation. Strengthening the back muscles can help prevent disk dislocation. See page 14.

 SARVANGASANA (SHOULDERSTAND)

Particularly strategic to the support of the sympathetic and parasympathetic nervous systems, which make up the autonomic nervous system. In addition, by increasing blood flow to the scalp and brain, this pose has been clinically observed to promote vitality and increase memory, IQ and hair growth. Nerves from the brain go to every tissue of the body. Therefore, the body is dependent upon on the health of the brain and spine. See page 17.

Clinical Benefits
By increasing circulation to the cranial tissues and organs, the Shoulderstand builds up a healthy brain and tones the entire nervous system. In addition it strengthens all the endrocrine glands, in particular the pineal gland (which produces the hormone melatonin), helping to balance the sympathetic (active) and parasympathetic (relaxed) nervous system as well as the pituitary, thyroid and parathyroid glands. Balancing the nervous system and increasing circulation help to strengthen the prostate gland in men and the uterus in women. The entire nervous system is strengthened,

helping to improve memory, depression, anxiety and other nervous disorders. The digestive and genitourinary systems are also strengthened.

CAVEAT: If you need to cough, swallow or sneeze while in the pose, come down, or you may gag or choke. Avoid this pose if you have a fever, headache or neurologic disturbance in the cranial viscera (tissues and organs of the brain).

❀ MATSYASANA (FISH POSE) ❀

Extends the muscles of the neck and shoulders back, helping to increase the space between vertebrae, allowing them to breathe and alleviating any stress in these areas. It also increases circulation into the brain stem and the cranial nerves. It should always follow the Shoulderstand. See page 20.

Yoga Nidra (Deep Relaxation)

By progressively releasing tension from each part of the body and increasing circulation, by contracting and releasing the muscles, yoga nidra helps restore the natural health of the body's entire nervous system. When you are lying in the supine position, all of the nerves and vertebrae that support the spine are allowed to "let go" and completely relax, helping to promote normal spinal alignment. I have used this practice with my private patients as an adjunct treatment for migraines, in many cases clinically noted to be caused by stress and poor circulation. When my good friend Buffy Stewart was in post-op recovery from her brain tumor, I went to the hospital on a daily basis for a week and did the deep relaxation with her. It helped to relieve her headaches and the emotional trauma she was experiencing in the aftermath of surgery. It also enabled her to sleep, further promoting her recovery. See page 24.

Pranayama: Breathing Techniques

❀ DEERGHA SWASAM (DEEP BREATHING) ❀

Just by doing the deep breathing you're bringing increased oxygen (prana) into the brain, alleviating vascular tension and constriction, thereby promoting mental vitality and reducing mental stress and fatigue. The oxygen you fill your entire lungs with permeates throughout the body, into all the nerve plexes and cells. See page 27.

❀ KAPALA BATHI (SKULL SHINING) ❀

Because of the vitality and energy produced by the vigorous repetition of breaths, the entire nervous system is both revitalized and strengthened. See page 28.

❀ NADDI SUDDHI (NERVE PURIFICATION) ❀

By relaxing, purifying and strengthening the subtle nerve currents along the spine and in the brain, *Naddi Suddhi* helps prevent memory loss and restore memory as well as reduces mental and emotional stress. It is strategically effective in diffusing the effects of negative emotions such as anger, fear and anxiety. Try it sometime. When you're in the throes of an anxious or difficult moment, or are caught up in an angry response, walk away from the aggravation. If your significant other, friend, family member or coworker has pushed a sensitive button, if you just got a parking ticket or, worse yet, your car has been towed, take a few moments and do this practice. You'll be surprised how immediate the therapeutic result can be. It can feel as though a dark cloud of stress has lifted from you. The more you do it, the more its strengthening effects build up in your system so you're less likely to get aggravated in the first place. When done in combination with the other asanas in this model and the thirty-minute Yoga for Health Practice Set I (pages 3–30) on a regular basis, the results can be life-changing. See page 28.

Advanced Asana

SIRHASANA (HEADSTAND)

Because of the difficulty level of this pose, please ensure that you are proficient with the Yoga for Health Practice Set I (pages 3–30) before attempting it. Only more advanced yoga practitioners should perform it, and under the supervision of a certified yoga instructor in the beginning. Avoid doing this pose if you have a medical condition related to the brain, neck or spine, or if you have a fever or headache.

The Headstand involves seven stages. Practice stages 1 to 3 for the first few days to build up strength and balance. Then you may progress to stages 4 to 6 and practice for a few days before moving on.

Stage 1: Kneel. Lock your fingers and create an angle on the floor with your forearms in front of you. Your locked fingers serve as the vertex of the angle. The distance between your elbows should be a forearm's length, thus forming an equilateral triangle.

Stage 2: Place the crown of your head on the floor, close to your locked fingers, so that your locked fingers are supporting the back of your head.

Stage 3: Slowly lift your trunk, bringing it perpendicular to the ground. In order to do this you need to raise your knees and bring your toes in, toward your face. When you have raised your trunk sufficiently, you will automatically feel that your toes can lift slowly off the ground, without any jumping or jerking. Conversely, if your trunk is not lifted sufficiently, and if your toes are jerked up, you may fall backward.

Stage 4: After getting used to the earlier stages of the Headstand, you can now move on. Slowly lift your toes and fold your legs so that your heels come closer to your buttocks, with the soles of your feet facing upward.

Stage 5: Gently lift your thighs, bringing them through a horizontal position.

Stage 6: Slowly straighten and align your thighs with your trunk. Keep your spine erect. Your knees will now face up and your legs will be hanging down behind your thighs.

Practice stages 4 through 6 until you have established an easy, steady balance in them.

Stage 7: Now you're ready to complete the pose. Make sure of your balance in stages 4 through 6 before progressing. Little by little, unfold your legs upward to form the full pose. Your bodyweight should be allowed to fall onto the top of the head, with your forearms placed lightly on the floor only to maintain balance.

Hold for ten seconds in the beginning and increase incrementally according to capacity. Come out of the pose if you have to cough, swallow or sneeze to avoid choking.

Clinical Benefits

The Headstand strengthens the brain and strengthens and tones the entire nervous system. It reinforces the immune function by strengthening the endrocrine glands, including the pineal and pituitary glands situated in the center of the brain, the thyroid and parathyroid in the throat and the thymus gland above the heart (helping in the circulation of white blood cells). It strengthens the prostate gland as well as the uterus and ovaries. It nourishes and fortifies the seminal fluid.

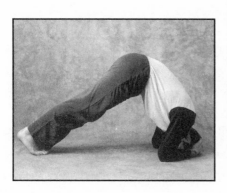
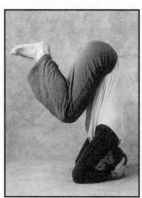
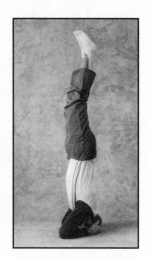

The Gastrointestinal System

PRIMARY ORGANS

Large intestine

Small intestine

Liver

Gallbladder

Pancreas

Stomach

Related disease conditions

Ulcers

Irritable bowel syndrome

Constipation

Diverticulitis

Appendicitis

Cirrhosis

Diarrhea

Gastritis

Hemorrhoids

Hepatitis, viral

Pancreatitis

The primary organs of the gastrointestinal system are the stomach and the small and large intestine (colon). However, this system is reliant upon the health of the gallbladder, the pancreas and the liver as well as on the proper balance of the sympathethic (active) and parasympathetic (relaxation) nervous systems for proper functioning. By promoting circulation and dispersing congestion in the organs of this system, the asanas in this section are particularly beneficial in enhancing and restoring their health, proving effective in both preventing and treating gastrointestinal disease and discomfort.

Recommended Asanas

❀ BHUJANGASANA (COBRA POSE) ❀

Provides a gentle massage to the abdomen. According to clinical studies, this pose increases pressure within the stomach (measured in millimeters of mercury, it produces the equivalent to 40–50 mm of mercury). The kidneys and adrenal glands are also massaged, improving circulation and helping to prevent stone formation. See page 9.

❀ SALABHASANA (LOCUST POSE) ❀

Massages your abdomen (increased abdominal pressure to the tune of 70–80 mm of mercury has been recorded). This pose also strengthens the front abdominal muscles and promotes support of the spine. It slims and tones your waistline by the gentle pressure being applied to the abdominal fascia (connective tissue in the muscles). Because it massages the digestive tract, moving the food along, this pose is particularly effective in preventing constipation. In addition, the resulting increase in circulation means a greater exchange of nutrients for waste products, leading to healthier-looking skin. See page 11.

CAVEAT: It is imperative not to go beyond your level of comfort when doing this pose. The Locust is soothing and beneficial only if you do not strain. Anyone with lower back pain should consult with a physician before doing this pose. It's not recommended for anyone with vertebral disk pathology.

Lie facedown with your chin against the floor. Tuck your arms beneath your body, palms up, beneath your thighs. Try to make your elbows touch. Keep your toes pointed. Inhale and retain the breath. Stiffen your body and raise both legs without bending your knees. Allow your weight to rest on your chest and arms. Hold for approximately ten seconds. When coming out of this pose, slowly lower your legs and release the breath.

> *Sweet remembrancer!—*
> *Now, good digestion wait on appetite,*
> *And health on both!*
>
> —William Shakespeare

🌼 DHANYURASANA (BOW POSE) 🌼

Massages and draws blood to the abdominal organs. Stomach pressure has been shown to increase by 50–60 mm of mercury, and direct pressure is applied to the liver, gallbladder, spleen and pancreas as well. The kidneys and adrenals also receive a massage. Once you are comfortable in the pose, you can begin a gentle rocking, propelled by the breath, which will increase the abdominal massage effect.

What is commonly called the "solar" plexus corresponds anatomically with the "celiac plexus," found in the middle of the abdomen. This plexus provides nerve supply to the digestive system and contains fibers from the parasympathetic nervous system that promote digestion. This posture stimulates parasympathetic action.

Lie facedown with your forehead against the floor. Bring your heels into your buttocks and reach back. Keeping your arms straight, grasp your feet, ankles or lower calves. Inhale and gently raise your head, chest and thighs off the floor. Arch your back and allow the entire weight of your body to rest on your abdomen. Hold the breath.

To come out of this pose, exhale slowly as you release your legs and slowly lower your chest and head to the floor. Turn your head to the side and relax in Savasana (see page 9) with your arms alongside your body.

Because this is a somewhat strenuous pose and requires flexibility in the legs, the beginner should perform it in stages. First, keep your forehead on the floor and just see if you can grasp your ankles or lower calves. If there is a lot of tension or if you feel the strain, allow your legs to relax with your heels against your buttocks. This stretches your thighs and calves. Then, if possible, straighten your arms and gently raise your thighs. If you can, raise your head and chest off the floor. If you need to, gradually work into the pose little by little each day. As your legs become more flexible, you can begin raising your head and chest. Be patient with yourself. Hold for approximately five to eight seconds.

CAVEAT: Do not pull your legs up by bending your elbows. Keep your arms straight. Anyone with acute back symptomatology, high blood pressure, a hernia or an ulcer in the stomach or intestines should avoid doing this pose.

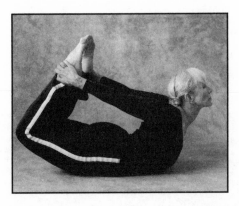

JANUSIRASANA (HEAD-TO-KNEE POSE)

This forward-bending posture stimulates and massages the parasympathetic nervous system, which has sensors in the lower spine. Massaging these fibers produces a relaxation effect that feels good. Systemically, it promotes circulation to the lower bowel, helping to prevent constipation and hemorrhoids. The increased blood supply can help the body repair the muscles and lining of the bowel, while the gentle pressure facilitates the movement of food along the digestive tract. Since it directly stimulates the parasympathetic nervous system, it causes the contents of the bowel to move along more effectively. See page 14.

❈ PASCHIMOTHANASANA (FULL FORWARD BEND) ❈

The Full Forward Bend stimulates, massages and relaxes the pelvic floor muscles. Lie on your back. Stretch your arms over your head, if you can do so comfortably, and lock your thumbs. Slowly raise your arms, head and chest, sitting in an upright position. If you find this too difficult, just sit up comfortably, then raise your arms above your head.

Slowly bend forward over your legs as far as you can comfortably go. Grasp your legs wherever you can reach comfortably—your ankles, calves or thighs. Relax your face into your knees if you are able to. Otherwise, relax your head to your chest. Relax in this position, breathing normally, for ten seconds. Do not bend your knees.

When coming out of this pose, lock your thumbs and stretch out over your legs, then rise into an upright position. Bring your hands to your lap and lie back comfortably in a supine position.

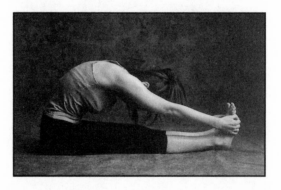

❈ SARVANGASANA (SHOULDERSTAND) ❈

Hemorrhoids result when the constant pressure of gravity exceeds what the valves in the veins can handle. Regular practice of the Shoulderstand can provide both a preventive measure and relief from this condition. See page 17.

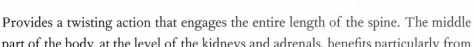
Provides a twisting action that engages the entire length of the spine. The middle part of the body, at the level of the kidneys and adrenals, benefits particularly from this. Increased pressure in the stomach of 30–40 mm of mercury has been measured.

Sit on the floor and bring your knees to your chest. Extend your right leg straight up. Cross your right foot over your left knee, placing the sole of your right foot flat on the floor. Sitting up straight, bring your right knee close to your chest. Now extend your arms in front of you, locking your thumbs and twisting to the right. Unlock your thumbs and place your right hand on the floor behind you, close to your body, with your fingers pointing away from you. Place your left arm between your trunk and your right knee (i.e., on the outside of your right knee) and press your knee to the right. You can also wrap your left arm around your right knee, bringing it close to your chest. Slowly twist your head and trunk to the right and look over your right shoulder. Hold for ten seconds. Then slowly unwind, coming back to center. Bring both knees to your chest, then repeat the pose with your left leg.

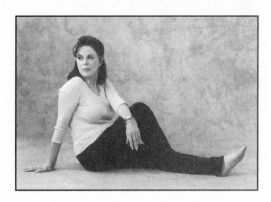

YOGA MUDRA (YOGIC SEAL)

Referred to in H.H. Sri Swami Satchidananda's *Integral Yoga Hatha* as "the symbol of Yoga," this is considered a very powerful pose that should finish any session of postures. It stimulates the parasympathetic nervous system, in the lower spine, helping to produce a profound sensation of relaxation, and increases stomach pressure by 20 mm of mercury. The heels contact the lower bowel, massaging it and helping to prevent or alleviate constipation.

Sit on the floor in a comfortable cross-legged position. Place your hands behind your back and grasp your right wrist with your left hand. Inhale, slowly bend forward and touch the floor with your forehead first and then, gradually, your chin. If you have only a limited range of motion, just relax forward as far as you can and relax your chin to your chest. The focus is the center of your forehead. On the exhalation, stretch your chin out and slowly rise.

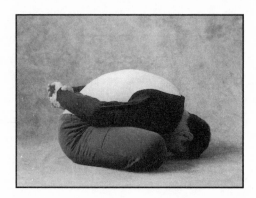

Pranayama (Breathing Practices)

❀ DEERGA SWASAM (DEEP BREATHING) ❀

This type of breathing massages the abdominal organs and the digestive tract, improving circulation and thus assisting the gastrointestinal system in achieving optimal nutrition, maintenance and repair. See page 27.

✿ KAPALA BATHI (SKULL SHINING) ✿

Massages the abdominal organs. It helps prevent constipation and other abdominal complaints by increasing circulation and energy in that region. Repeat three times. See page 28.

✿ NADDI SUDDHI (NERVE PURIFICATION) ✿

Balances the sympathetic (active) and parasympathetic (relaxing) nervous systems, producing a calming effect. By calming the nervous system, alternate nostril breathing helps prevent the nervous discharge of energy. Thus the gastrointestinal tract receives an increase in blood supply, which spikes the appetite. Because of the relative increase in circulation, the gastrointestinal tract can work more efficiently. Practice for five minutes. See page 28.

Advanced Asana

✿ MAYURASANA (PEACOCK POSE) ✿

Before attempting the Peacock Pose you must be completely proficient in the Yoga for Health Practice Set I on pages 3–30. It is intended only for those more advanced in their practice of Hatha yoga. Because of the degree of difficulty involved, your body needs to be strengthened and prepared for the physical dynamics involved in performing this pose. It should not be done by anyone with gastrointestinal or lower-back conditions.

Stage 1: In a kneeling position, place the palms together on the floor, with the fingers pointing toward the knees. There should be a forearm's length between the fingers and the knees. Slowly bend the body forward, bending the arms first. Rest the forehead on the floor. In this position, the chest is supported by the upper arms, and the stomach rests against the joined elbows. Stretch the legs out behind you, with the toes resting on the floor. Raise the head. Stiffen the entire body like a bar resting on a fulcrum. Practice this first stage until you have your strength and balance and can do it easily.

Stage 2: Gently move the entire body forward with the help of the toes, thereby shifting the entire weight of the body toward the head. When the upper and lower halves of the body are in balance, the toes will automatically rise off the floor. To come out of the posture, first place the toes on the floor and then the knees. Rest in a kneeling position, sitting back on your heels.

The Peacock Pose strengthens all the musculature in the body. It strengthens the abdominal (oblique) muscles and the abdominal viscera (small intestine and colon). The applied pressure to the abdominal bowl by the elbows increases circulation into the abdominal viscera and aids in the function of digestion and the prevention of constipation. It also helps to alleviate emotional stress in the solar plexus located in the abdominal plexus.

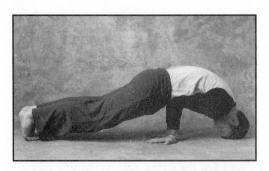

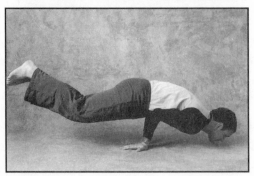

The Immune System

PRIMARY ORGANS

Bone marrow

Thymus

Spleen

Lymph nodes

Liver

Related disease conditions

Cancer

Allergies

Fibromyalgia

Hepatitis

Arthritis

Juvenile diabetes

Diabetes

Rheumatoid arthritis

Multiple sclerosis

Chronic fatigue

Chron's disease

Anemia

Addison's disease

The body's immune system is central to its overall health. It detects invaders and protects the body and its organs and systems from them, whether they are toxins or disease-causing agents such as bacteria and viruses. When functioning properly, the immune system prevents chronic diseases, fights infections and increases longevity.

There are two primary ways the immune system begins to malfunction. First, by overreacting to a substance that normally isn't a threat, such as pollen, causing an allergic reaction, or to substances that cause arthritis or lupus. Second, it can weaken and fail to react appropriately, thus allowing the growth of cancerous cells, the spread of herpes viruses or the development of conditions such as chronic fatigue syndrome. It also predisposes the system to less serious conditions such as colds and the flu.

> *Man is an intelligence in servitude to his organs.*
> —ALDOUS HUXLEY

The major organs of the immune system are dispersed throughout the body. They include the lymph nodes (situated in groups along lymphatic vessels), bone marrow (in the core of bones), the thymus (in the upper part of the chest) and the spleen (on the left side of the abdomen). These organs produce and store an array of white blood cells and specialized immune cells. These cells help the body detect invading agents, produce antibodies that neutralize or destroy them, turn off the immune reaction when it is no longer needed and store the process in their memory for future reference.

The yoga asanas that follow balance and promote circulation into the specific glands and organs that can then more efficiently do their work.

Recommended Asanas

SARVANGASANA (SHOULDERSTAND)

Lymph fluids circulate via small channels that contain one-way valves. Lymph reenters the bloodstream beneath the left collarbone, where it is processed through the liver, spleen and kidneys—organs that are vital in keeping the immune system strong and healthy.

Nearly the entire column of blood and lymph must rise against gravity in order to circulate. By placing the body in the Shoulderstand, circulation of the lymph is significantly enhanced. The pineal and pituitary glands that balance the sympathetic and parasympathetic nervous systems are reinforced. The thymus and thyroid glands are regulated. And the pancreas, liver and spleen receive an increased blood supply, thereby further supporting the immune system. See page 17.

MATSYASANA (FISH POSE)

Increases the volume of air in the lungs. It is clinically useful for the prevention and treatment of bronchitis, asthma and other chronic lung complaints. It also lowers blood pressure because it stimulates the baroreceptors (stretch receptors) in the neck. The baroreceptors send signals to the central nervous system in proportion to the mean (steady) blood pressure and rate of change of blood pressure within respective vessels, resulting in a relaxation response. See page 20.

> *There used to be a real me . . . but then I had it surgically removed.*
>
> —PETER SELLERS

ARDDHAMATSYANDRASANA (HALF SPINAL TWIST)

The twisting action of the spinal column works on the entire spine to relieve muscular strain, backache and neckache. In addition, massagelike pressure is applied to the kidneys, liver, gallbladder and pancreas. When the pancreas, which produces insulin, is functioning properly because of optimum circulation, it can self-regulate more effectively, proving beneficial in the prevention and treatment of diabetes. See page 22.

Yoga Nidra (Deep Relaxation)

As discussed in the cardiovascular section, by letting go of tension, by contracting and releasing the body parts and slowing the breath, the body enters into a much deeper state of relaxation, measured to be even more restful than a good night's sleep. This deep state of relaxed awareness lowers blood pressure, removes stressful impediments from the natural healthy circulation of the blood and lymph and allows all of the body's primary glands and organs that affect the immune system to rebalance themselves.

As Dr. Herbert Benson discovered in his studies on meditation, through deep relaxation practice blood sugar and diabetes control are significantly affected, and thyroid function (whether too low or too high) is stabilized. All of this helps in the healthy function of the immune system.

Dr. Benson and others from Harvard Medical School have also found that meditation and relaxation techniques slow the metabolic rate to a pace where the cells actually require less oxygen because they aren't working as hard. It often takes several hours of sleep to reach the level of refreshment obtained by just a few minutes of deep relaxation.

Please refer to Part II (pages 87–208) for elaboration on the use of this practice in the treatment of cancer and other immune-related diseases.

Your body is perfectly still but your mind is loose and on its own. In hyperdrive . . . You might suddenly start wondering about random, unexpected, unusual or even very ordinary things. About parallel parking. The sexual orientation of your cat. Or your own. What to have for dinner. Where Dick Cheney is. David Letterman's hair . . . No matter what subject comes up, the trick is to keep watching and creating a distance between you and these random thoughts. Ultimately, you will find that none of the chatter matters. In the perfect present moment of your meditation, all that matters is that you go beyond the worries, differences and everyday thoughts so you can recover from their effects on you. So you can continue enjoying the everyday drama and minutiae of your life.

If a thought persists to the point that you're compelled to stop your meditation, try making a deal with your mind. Make a mental note and tell it you'll give it your

> *I'm married with one son and the sole proprietor of an auto body shop that caters to celebrities and corporate accounts. It's been stressful down the road to my business's success. In my early thirties I began having lower back discomfort and difficulty concentrating on my work due to all the responsibilities of family and work. Then I was introduced to Swami Satchidananda's method of Integral Yoga as a form of yoga therapy to help reduce my back pain and stress. I began doing the postures, relaxation (yoga nidra) and breathing techniques every night. Day by day I began to watch my stress levels and angry responses to aggravating situations lessen. I began dealing with my daily problems more effectively. Practicing yoga has helped me get through the physical and emotional difficulties of my life. I wish I had known about it when I was younger.*
>
> —KOREY TATAYAN, MID-THIRTIES, OWNER/MANAGER, BON VOYAGE AUTO BODY SHOP, SANTA MONICA, CALIFORNIA

undivided attention when the session ends. I've done this in my practice many times. If you keep at it and don't give in, your mind will eventually surrender and relax into a more neutral state. This has been proven many times over, even in the most difficult cases. This is where you begin experiencing the empirical medical benefits of the practice of meditation.

When your subjective mind and ego step aside, your system can respond to the mechanisms of the practice that will bring your blood pressure back to normal, strengthen your immune system and stabilize the sinus rhythm of the heart. In this way your system can actually experience the medical benefits described in Part II that Drs. Benson, Ornish, Pacia and others talk about in the medical studies that verify that yoga and meditation can reverse heart disease and treat other acute and chronic diseases. When we reach this place in meditation, beyond all the differences, conditions and conflicts of politics, relationships, race, religion, sexual orientation and fashion, we not only prevent but let go of the causes of our disease and adverse conditions. We experience the oneness in us all. We begin healing, not only ourselves but our relationships and the whole world.

> *Life is a tragedy when seen in close-up, but a comedy in the long run.*
> —Charles Chaplin

As you begin your practice, sit in a comfortable cross-legged position. Place a small pillow beneath the coccyx (the back part of the buttocks) to slant the legs downward. If it's uncomfortable to sit in this position unsupported—and for many it will be—try any of the following:

- sit against a wall with your legs outstretched
- sit in a chair
- if you're in poor health, meditate while lying in bed.

In other words, there is never an excuse not to meditate. Meditation can be practiced anywhere—in your office, on the beach, in a dentist's chair. The important thing to remember is that it should be done on a regular basis, every day, to achieve maximum results.

In order to create the right atmosphere, begin your session with three "oms," followed by the pranayama (breathing practices). Do at least three rounds of Kapala

Bathi (see page 28) first. Follow this with five minutes of Naddi Suddhi (see page 28). As you progress in your practice, increase your Kapala Bathi to five minutes and the Naddi Suddhi to fifteen, or as long as is comfortable.

One very effective meditation technique is the "mantra meditation." A mantra is a sound construct that produces a very relaxing sensation in the mind and the nervous system. It contains a "peaceful and healing vibration" or energy that resonates in the energy centers of the body called "chakras." There are universal mantras such as "Om Shanthi" or "Hari Om" that the beginner can use. "Hari Om" is the first mantra I used. I was experiencing a lot of tension in my abdominal plexus, or "solar plexus," a part of the body that is considered its "emotional center," and in my throat. The "Hari Om" mantra brought me a lot of relief by relieving the buildup of stress in those areas. The "ha" sound emanates from the abdomen, the "ri" resonates in the throat and the "om" in the pineal gland (situated in the center of the brain). The pineal gland thereby releases the hormone melatonin into the nervous system.

The word *Amen* is considered a mantra; the name of sacred prophets can be used, such as Allah or Jehovah or Waken Tanken (a Native American deity). Each of these holy names contains a vibration or energy that, when pronounced, resonates in the nervous system, producing a very peaceful and harmonious sensation in the mind and body. When a person finds a guru whose teachings they are comfortable with, it is customary for the guru to provide the student with a personal mantra. Whatever mantra you end up using, it's the repetition of the sound on a regular basis that will benefit your practice of meditation.

After repeating your mantra for several minutes, your mind begins to settle into the "feeling" or "vibration." You can just sit and allow your mind and body to experience the peaceful quality that results. Some practi-

I began to practice yoga when I was fifteen. I took a class in high school as an alternative to other PE classes such as weight training and modern dance. At first I felt somewhat self-conscious about my practice; there were many people in the class who were particularly flexible, and our teacher spoke more about what a pose should look like than about the process and individual aspect of our bodies and minds. I tried really hard to get my heels to the floor, my back straight, my arms curved around, etc., and in all honesty, I found the class more frustrating than enlightening.

That summer, I started to do yoga on my own. I would go to a flat rock by the lighthouse where I live to do my poses as the fishing boats went by. I wouldn't worry about how I looked or how stiff I was because each day my experience was different. That was the real beginning of my yoga practice. I discovered that, for me, yoga was the purity of the practice, not the attainment of a pose's perfection.

—WILLA MAMET, UNDERGRADUATE STUDENT, BROWN UNIVERSITY, PROVIDENCE, RHODE ISLAND

tioners begin to see lights and images. Some hear sounds of various frequencies. Others may experience a calm and centering sensation within the mind and body. All these experiences share equal value. Just relax into the experience. As you do, you'll find that it gives you a deeper, more expanded experience of yourself. It will connect you to a larger understanding of life and the entire universe, enabling the experience of unity with all living beings, all things. All the labels and definitions we place on each other and on ways of life fall away. Meditation takes you into neutral realms of peace and love you never dreamed possible. There are no words to describe it.

> *Where there is love, there is life.*
> —MAHATMA GANDHI

Most important, the calming, centering and transcendental experience of meditation will dynamically influence the way you interact with every aspect of your daily life—your relationships with others and with yourself, shopping for groceries, driving in heavy traffic, absorbing world and domestic crises, playing tennis, writing a book, directing a film, being alone. With the influence of meditation, every moment will begin to bring you closer to you. As my guru teaches, ultimately your life itself will become a meditation.

In the Resources section you'll find a comprehensive guide of books and audio products on meditation that will further support your practice.

Pranayama: Breathing Techniques

DEERGA SWASAM (DEEP BREATHING)

When your breathing slows and becomes deeper and more rhythmical, your heart rate slows and blood pressure drops. Muscle tension eases. All of this contributes to balancing the sympathetic and parasympathetic nervous systems, and contributes to the support of the immune system. See page 27.

✿ KAPALA BATHI (SKULL SHINING) ✿

Enhances the body's immune function by oxygenating and strengthening the blood. It balances the sympathetic and parasympathetic nervous systems and increases "prana," vital energy, into all the glands and organs. See page 28.

✿ NADDI SUDDHI (NERVE PURIFICATION) ✿

By purifying the subtle currents in the spine and the brain, and balancing the sympathetic and parasympathetic nervous systems, alternate nostril breathing further supports the body's glands and organs. The combination of pranayama practices with the prescribed asanas strengthens and restores the immune system. See page 28.

The Endocrine System

PRIMARY ORGANS

Pineal gland

Pituitary gland

Thyroid gland

Pancreas

Liver

Spleen

Kidneys

Adrenal glands

Prostate gland

Uterus

Related disease conditions

AIDS

Prostate cancer

Ovarian cancer

Diabetes

Leukemia

Breast cancer

Obesity

Hasimoto's thyroiditis (underactive thyroid)

Graves' disease (overactive thyroid)

Urinary tract disease

A wide variety of physiological processes are carried out unconsciously by the endocrine system through chemical messengers called "hormones." The endocrine system is a collection of glands that produce these hormones, which are necessary for normal bodily functions. The hormones regulate metabolism, growth and sexual development. These glands release hormones directly into the bloodstream, where they are transported to organs and tissues throughout the body.

The most vital glands of this system are the pituitary, pineal, thyroid, adrenal, pancreas and sex glands. The pituitary and pineal glands are situated in the brain. The thyroid is in the neck region, the adrenals and pancreas in the solar plexus (abdominal) area and the sex glands in the pelvic region.

The yoga stretches included in this section optimize circulation through the endocrine glands. This enables them to perform more effectively in their maintenance and repair functions. Any inflammation, under- or overactive functioning or hormone imbalance can be most efficiently addressed by the body's self-regulatory mechanisms. Related disease conditions such as infec-

What we feel and think and are is to a great extent determined by the state of our ductless glands and viscera.

—ALDOUS HUXLEY

tion, AIDS and cancer may also be more appropriately tackled by the immune system when circulatory enhancement and rebalancing of the body's nervous systems of excitement and relaxation (sympathetic and parasympathetic) take place efficiently.

Recommended Asanas

✿ BHUJANGASANA (COBRA POSE) ✿

Stretching of the thyroid gland, at the base of the throat, provides a gentle massage that affects both blood supply and lymph flow. According to Dr. McLanahan and Dr. Ornish, the Cobra Pose in tandem with the Shoulderstand can be effective in correcting both an underactive and overactive thyroid. Dr. K. N. Udupa conducted research corroborating the normalizing effect of this pose on thyroid activity. See page 9.

✿ SARVANGASANA (SHOULDERSTAND) ✿

Stimulates the thyroid gland at the base of the throat, helping to stabilize the metabolism and prevent thyroid disease. It stimulates the pineal and pituitary glands in the center of the brain and rebalances the sympathetic and parasympathetic nervous systems—vitally important in supporting the endocrine system. See page 17.

✿ MATSYASANA (FISH POSE) ✿

By stretching the neck backward with the head on the floor, the Fish Pose applies pressure to the base of the throat, increasing circulation and balancing the thyroid gland—thereby helping to stabilize the metabolism. It should always follow the Shoulderstand to relieve tension in the throat, neck and upper back. See page 20.

ARDDHAMATSYANDRASANA (HALF SPINAL TWIST)

The twisting motion of this pose applies pressure to the adrenal glands, situated in the mid back. These glands produce a variety of hormones, such as adrenaline and cortisone, essential for controlling stress and enhancing immunity. It also causes them to release extra energy, and boosts vitality. The twisting activity also increases circulation to the kidneys, pancreas and spleen, helping to reduce stress and rebalance these glands and organs. See page 22.

The Spinal-Skeletal/Musculo-Ligamentous System

AREAS AFFECTED

Cervical spine

Cervical paraspinals

Trapezius muscles

Thoracic spine

Intercostal muscles

Supraspinatus muscle

Infraspinatus muscle

Scapula

Teres muscle

Teres minor

Upper extremities

Deltoid bursa

Brachioradialis

Carpal

Lumbar spine

Erector spinae muscles

Quadradus luborum

Iliolumbar spine

Piriformis muscle

Gluteus muscles

Related disease conditions

General tightness of the fascia of the neck,
  mid and lower back

Arthritis

Muscular strain

Temporomandibular joint syndrome (TMJ)

Frozen shoulder syndrome

Bursitis

Kyphosis (rounding of the upper spine)

Lordosis (inversion of the lower spine)

Osteoporosis

Carpal tunnel syndrome

Sciatica

Low-back syndrome

The musculoskeletal system provides form, stability and movement to the human body. It consists of the body's bones (which make up the skeleton), muscles, tendons, ligaments, joints, cartilage and other connective tissue. The "connective tissue" (fascia) is the fibrous tissue that binds other tissues and organs together. Its chief components are elastic fibers and collagen, a protein substance. Connective tissue provides support to the various structures of the body, holding organs in place and providing the underlying structure for all tissues.

Yoga asanas stretch, massage and promote circulation, mobility and vitality in this system and all its components. The stretching of the joints in the asanas produces secretion of synovial fluid, a lubricant released into the joints that keeps them supple and removes waste products. The result is to reduce stiffness, which prevents arthritis and other joint-related conditions.

According to Dr. David Bozentka, assistant professor of orthopedic surgery at the University of Pennsylvania, a study conducted with a group of fifty-one patients diagnosed with carpal tunnel syndrome (CTS) showed significant improvements in pain and grip strength after eight weeks of specific Hatha yoga poses that focused on upper-body stretching and relaxation techniques. Dr. Bozentka theorizes that, in addition to the soft-tissue component involved, there is a psychosocial stress component that contributes to the condition. He believes that yoga relaxation and meditation play significant roles in alleviating these factors.

> *Why isn't there a special name for the tops of your feet?*
> —LILY TOMLIN

Recommended Asanas

❀ SURYA NAMASKARA (SUN SALUTATION) ❀

Provides a complete preventive therapy for the entire spine and increases circulation to all the joints and muscles. It is particularly recommended for prevention of carpal tunnel syndrome (CTS). See page 6.

❀ BHUJANGASANA (COBRA POSE) ❀

Recommended as a preventive measure for the upper spine, this pose helps to reverse the "kyphosis," or rounding of the thoracic spine (upper back). Kyphotic syndrome can gradually develop through the years as a result of poor posture. Many people who spend long hours at the computer or in professions that require prolonged sitting, bending and stooping are prone to this condition. The Cobra Pose strengthens the lower back muscles, helping the thoracic spine maintain its normal healthy alignment. By extending the head and spine up and back gently in a sustained manner, the rounding syndrome of the thoracic spine is gradually reversed. The Cobra stimulates the cranial nerves, relieving stress and giving a boost to both mental and physical energy. See page 9.

CAVEAT: Be careful to keep the elbows bent while doing this pose. Straightening the arms will strain the trapezius muscles and the intercostal fascia (the fibrous membrane connecting the ribs).

ARDHASALABASANA (HALF LOCUST)

Recommended for strengthening the lumbar spine (lower back) muscles and vertebrae. See page 10.

JANUSIRASANA (HEAD-TO-KNEE POSE)

Recommended for stretching and strengthening the lumbar paraspinals. It stretches the hamstring muscles behind the knees and stretches and strengthens the femoral muscles. It stretches the piriformis muscles in the buttocks and promotes circulation in the wrists, which helps prevent and treat carpal tunnel syndrome. See page 14.

SARVANGASANA (SHOULDERSTAND)

Promotes alignment of the vertebrae. See page 17.

HALASANA (PLOW POSE)

Similar to the Forward Bend, the Plow stimulates the parasympathetic nervous system, this time by way of the portion of this system located in the neck. The Plow is effective in releasing tight shoulder muscles as well as the muscles along the vertebral column of the neck. An increase in blood supply, caused by the change in gravity, aids tissue and muscle repair and relaxation as well.

Once you're comfortable in the Plow Pose you can vary it by grasping your toes and rolling your spine back and forth gently. Bring yourself to a seated position and then slowly roll back. The muscles along the spine that hold the vertebrae and surrounding muscles in place are temporarily relieved of their tense holding positions and can deeply relax.

Lie flat on your back, keeping your hands alongside your body and palms to the floor. Hold the breath and slowly raise your legs to a ninety-degree angle. Then raise your hips and the lower part of your back, bringing your legs to a vertical position in relation to the floor. Exhale, slowly lower your legs over your head and touch the floor with your toes.

As a variation, walk your toes close to your head or far from your head.

To come out of the pose, slowly roll your spine to the floor vertebra by vertebra, providing your back muscles with a gentle massage. See page 16.

CAVEAT: Be careful not to strain in this pose. If there is strain, you could sprain your shoulder and neck muscles. As you lower your legs over your head, be careful not to shake your body or lose control of your legs. Hold for approximately ten seconds.

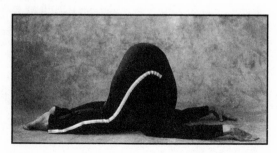

✿ MATSYASANA (FISH POSE) ✿

Recommended for preventive treatment of the upper spine. It helps to prevent kyphosis (rounding of the spine) associated with osteoporosis, age-related thinning of the bones and poor upper back posture often caused by prolonged sitting over a desk or laptop, and driving. It's clinically effective for the treatment of general upper back and shoulder tightness. See page 20.

✿ ARDDHAMATSYANDRASANA (HALF SPINAL TWIST) ✿

Recommended for preventive treatment of the upper and mid spine. It helps to alleviate tightness of the upper and mid back. I recommend it, as well as the Cobra, for my patients and students in professions that require sitting for prolonged periods of time. Take a few minutes, get out of your chair and do the poses. They will increase circulation into the fascia (connective tissue), relaxing your back so you can have a more comfortable day. See page 22.

✿ PAVANAMUKTASANA (WIND ELIMINATION) ✿

This pose is called Wind Elimination because, by massaging the digestive tract, it moves the contents along. If any gas has accumulated, it can be more efficiently expelled. In addition, the Wind Elimination is also an excellent way of relieving tension in the lower back by stretching and increasing circulation into the lumbar (lower back) muscles.

I use this pose effectively with my cardiac patients at Cedars-Sinai Medical Center to relieve tightness in that region immediately after performing the Shoulderstand. See page 21.

Yoga Nidra (Deep Relaxation)

See page 24.

With regard to supporting the spine, neck and back, deep relaxation quickly evokes a relaxation response in which blood pressure falls and breathing slows, allowing the body to rest. Our neck muscles work constantly while we are awake, holding up between ten and twelve pounds of head all day long. Our back muscles have to support the weight of the entire body. In deep relaxation these muscles can be at rest, allowing them the opportunity to let go of stress and stiffness.

CAVEAT: If you have pain in your neck and/or back, place a pillow under your knees and behind your head and neck as you lie in a supine position on the floor. If lying on the floor is uncomfortable, do this relaxation practice sitting in a chair or lying on your bed.

The Yoga Vitamin: A 10-Minute "Head-to-Toe" Micro-session

To Help Get You Through a Busy, Stressful Day

Strategic Benefits

* boosts immune function
* reduces stress
* increases vitality
* strengthens the cardiovasulcar system
* stabilizes blood pressure and metabolism

Whether you're at work, at school or on a business trip, find a quiet place for your yoga mat or a towel with enough room to do your postures, where you won't be interrupted for ten minutes.

I designed this time-effective micro program for several of my private yoga clients and patients in the film industry who fly around the world making movies or are on a regular soundstage shooting a TV series. No matter where they are or how busy their day, they can find the time to do their practice.

Although the asansas that make up this "yoga vitamin" are compressed into a short ten-minute session, they should be done slowly and with awareness and ease. As with the thirty-minute total health program, each posture is followed by a resting Savasana pose. This "yoga vitamin" is in no way intended to be a substitute for the complete Yoga for Health program.

The Program

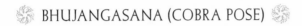

❁ BHUJANGASANA (COBRA POSE) ❁

= 30 SECONDS

The Cobra Pose applies pressure to the lungs and heart, encouraging an increase in lymph flow, which may help protect against heart disease. Some medical authorities feel that the flow of lymph may help determine how much plaque builds up in the coronary arteries.

To prepare, lie on your stomach in *Savasana* (Relaxation Pose), your arms alongside your body and your cheek to one side. Your legs should be about seventeen inches apart. Bring your forehead to the floor. Place your palms on the floor, below your shoulders, elbows raised and close to the trunk of your body. Relax all your muscles completely. Bring your legs close together with your toes pointed. Now slowly raise your head and bend your neck back as far as possible. Slowly raise your chest, bending your vertebrae backward one by one. Keep your elbows bent. Inhale while rising, relax into the pose and breathe normally. Exhale as you come down. Hold for ten seconds. Repeat.

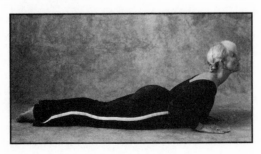

✿ SAVANGASANA (SHOULDERSTAND) ✿

= 3 MINUTES

With regard to the biochemical dynamic, the heart rate initially increases during the Shoulderstand, but then decreases below resting levels, producing a feeling of relaxation and calm. Resting your chin on your chest stimulates the pressure-sensitive "baroreceptors" in your neck, lowering blood pressure and pulse and thereby helping to relieve tension in the cardiovascular system.

With regard to circulation in general, the pull of gravity means that blood flow tends to pool in the legs and lower body. In the United States, a condition common among older people is swelling and discoloration in the legs and feet. Varicose veins and hemorrhoids result when the constant pull of gravity exceeds what the valves in the veins can handle. A daily Shoulderstand may act as a preventive technique for these and other circulatory-related conditions.

> *While filming* Dragnet *I would kick off my heels, get down on the floor and go into the ten-minute session that Nirmala gave me for my lungs and back. I would feel better. Really better. If we take a moment to take care of ourselves, we open up. Like a flower to the sun. We are more available to the day, to others. It's wonderful. Yoga is subtle and operates deeply, at the level of the breath. And the breath is life.*
>
> —LINDSAY CROUSE

Adjust your clothing to loosen any restrictions in movement. Lie on your back with your feet together and your arms alongside your body, palms down. Inhale, straighten your legs and lift them over your head in a horizontal position as shown in the illustration. (If necessary, bend your knees in order to raise them over your head.) Straighten your legs into a vertical position, keeping them together. Bring your palms to your lower back for support. Breathe normally. Keep your chin tucked into your chest. Hold for two minutes.

To come out of the pose, lower your legs over your head, parallel to the floor. Bring your arms to the floor to the posterior back for support. Slowly roll your spine to the floor, keeping your legs straight if you can. Otherwise, bend your knees as you come down. Continue breathing normally.

Relax in Savasana.

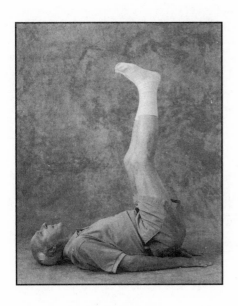
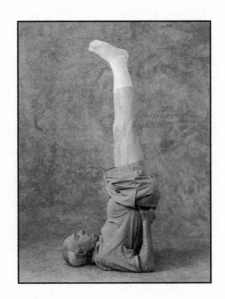

🌸 MATSYASANA (FISH POSE) 🌸

⚊ 30 SECONDS

The Fish Pose is a complementary pose to the Shoulderstand. Lie flat on the floor with your palms pressed against the sides of your thighs. Shift your bodyweight to your elbows and raise your head and trunk. Arch your chest, then lower the crown of your head to the floor, creating a bridge between your head and buttocks. Expand your chest as much as possible and bring a smile to your lips to break up tension in the jaw.

To come out of the pose, place your bodyweight on your elbows again and raise your head gently. Then slowly roll your spine to the floor. Deep breathing through the nose enhances the benefit of this practice. Do not hold your breath.

The Fish Pose stretches the thyroid, neck and shoulder muscles in the opposite direction to the Shoulderstand. Because it shortens the space between the posterior aspects of the vertebrae in the neck, it should be done very slowly. Try to stretch your neck out as you stretch it back. As I discuss later, this pose is used in clinical settings in the treatment of respiratory diseases.

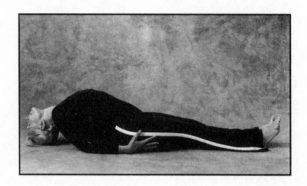

YOGA NIDRA (DEEP RELAXATION)

☰ 3 MINUTES

Lie on your back in a comfortable supine position with your arms and legs extended. Your legs should be about a foot and a half apart, and your arms a few inches away from the body with your palms up. Close your eyes and, breathing through your nose, begin relaxing into the position. Bring your awareness to your right leg and foot. Tense the leg. Lift it off the floor a few inches. Tense a little more and let it drop. Roll it from side to side and just forget about it. Repeat with the left leg.

Now inhale and tense your pelvis and buttocks. Squeeze the tension out. Most of us hold a lot of stress in this area, which can lead to disorders in the reproductive system as well as in the pelvis and hips. Now inhale and fill your stomach with air. Hold it for a few moments and then release through your mouth. Just let it gush out. Inhale again, fill your stomach with air. Then bring it into your chest. Hold it. Open your mouth and let it gush out. Experience the warm sensation of the release.

Bring your awareness to your right hand and arm. Inhale, close your hand into a gentle fist and begin tensing tightly all the way to your shoulder. Then release. Repeat with your left hand and arm.

Inhale and raise your shoulders to your ears. Hold for a moment. Then release. Turn your head from side to side, slowly. Then center and relax. Bring the awareness to your face. Open your mouth and drop your jaw. Move it from side to side. Then center and relax. Now tense your face into a tight prune face. And release. Open your mouth wide and extend your tongue as far as you can. And then relax. Your body should be completely relaxed and free of tension at this point.

To begin the second phase of the practice, without moving, bring your mental awareness to your feet. Begin mentally relaxing your feet. Now bring your mental awareness up your entire body, relaxing each part until you reach your head. Once your body is free of all stress, bring your mental awareness to your breath. At this point, when your breath is quite still, bring awareness to your mind. Begin watching your mind. Begin watching your thoughts as they enter and leave your mind. You most likely will find that your mind begins to fill with thoughts at this point, particularily if you are new to this practice. It's a common experience. The important thing is not to push the thoughts away. Don't force anything. Just continue watching the phenomenon as though you're watching a film. After doing this practice a few times you will find that eventually your mind will begin to relax and let go of the thoughts. Then you'll begin to experience a very relaxed, blissful quality within yourself.

Remain in this quiet place of detached relaxation and deep, calm awareness for a few moments. Then slowly bring your awareness back to the breath and let it gradually deepen. Imagine that you're breathing all the way into your feet. Let the awareness rise through your body, waking up all the parts until you reach your head. Then begin gently moving parts of your body. Observe the relaxed and easeful quality within them. Sit up and prepare for your pranayama (breathing practices).

Because much of its emphasis is on reducing stress, the deep relaxation is considered by physicians such as Dr. McLanahan and Dr. Ornish to be strategic in strengthening and supporting the cardiovascular system. The guided relaxation has been shown to affect both biochemical and nervous discharge in the direction of a more relaxed state. Blood pressure falls and breathing slows, allowing your heart to rest deeply. The process is physiologically more restful than a good night's sleep, yet takes only a few minutes.

Pranayama

❁ DEERGA SWASAM (DEEP BREATHING) ❁

= 1 MINUTE

Sit in a cross-legged position, using a wall for support if necessary. Your spine should be erect, your chest expanded with the shoulders and neck relaxed. Exhale completely. Inhale and fill your abdomen, then your rib cage, then bring the air into your chest. Exhale slowly from your chest, then rib cage, then abdomen.

Clinical Benefits
Besides maximizing oxygen intake into the blood and all of the nerves, organs and glands, deep breathing balances the parasympathetic nervous system (located in the lower back), supporting the function of the cardiovascular system and the immune system. Slow, deep, rhythmic breathing produces a feeling of relaxation and ease throughout the entire body and within the mind, helping you to recover from the effects of a stressful, hectic day.

❁ KAPALA BATHI (SKULL SHINING) ❁

= 1 MINUTE

This is an invigorating practice you can do without having to exert much physical energy. The only muscles doing the work are the abdominals (and those in the spine, if you're sitting in an unsupported position), thereby strengthening the back.

Exhale completely through your nose. Inhale and produce a quick contraction of your abdomen, expelling the air. Then inhale and expel the air again. Repeat rapidly seven or eight times. The inhalation and exhalation should have equal force. Have a long exhalation. Rest for a moment. Repeat three times.

Clinical Benefits

Kapala Bathi increases oxygen levels in the blood, helping to elevate your energy level. The heat produced in your system by doing this breathing burns waste products from the blood as well. It strengthens the parasympathetic nervous system, thereby reducing stress and creating a feeling of balance in your body and mind. By both relaxing and energizing your system, this dynamic breathing practice will help you get through any stressful day.

❋ NADDI SUDDHI (ALTERNATE NOSTRIL BREATHING) ❋

= 1 MINUTE

Sit in a comfortable cross-legged position. Make a loose fist with your right hand. Release your thumb and last two fingers. Relax your right arm against your chest and close your right nostril with your right thumb. Slowly exhale as much air as possible without strain through your left nostril. Then inhale through your left nostril and close it with the last two fingers of your right hand. Exhale through your right nostril.

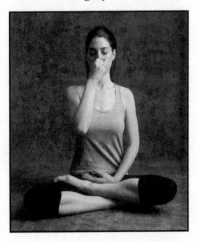

The results of this exercise have been clinically measured by EEG (electroencephalograph) and demonstrated to balance activity in the two hemispheres of the brain, which produces an increased sense of relaxation, necessary for the support of both the immune and cardiovascular systems. It is known to help stabilize the heart from arrythmias and restore equilibrium to the nervous system.

PART Two

Rehabilitation

Yoga for Health Practice Set II: A Restorative Yoga Program for the Treatment of Acute and Chronic Disease

NOTE: If you have been diagnosed with a specific condition, consult with your treating physician and a certified yoga therapist before doing this program or any of the poses included herein.

Based on the Hatha Yoga Cardiac Program at Cedars-Sinai Medical Center Preventive and Rehabilitative Cardiac Center, this program provides specific poses to include in your yoga practice to help you recover from various medical conditions.

The Yoga for Health restorative program is a variation of the "standard" beginning Yoga for Health program (in Part I) used by healthy practitioners with full flexibility. While for the most part the sequence of postures is the same, their practical application is modified to accommodate individuals with physical limitations and a restricted range of motion. Because the levels of difficulty are lower, the restorative program is less intimidating to patients who are restricted in their flexibility and range of motion.

In other words, patients who have a particular medical condition that prevents them from participating in the "standard" Yoga for Health program will find they can easily do the modified asanas in this restorative program with ease and confidence. If you aren't sure which format to use, consult with either your physician or a certified yoga therapist.

Many of my patients in the Cedars-Sinai Hatha Yoga cardiac program are in a postoperative phase, anywhere from one week to three months after surgery. At first some are intimidated about doing any kind of physical activity. However, they soon find they are able to do one or two poses. Because the effort required is minimal, they soon build up their strength and capacity to add poses. Both Dr. McLanahan and I recommend this program for anyone who is physically limited or disabled, or in a postoperative phase of recovery.

> *Anything you call "yours" is not you. You are the passenger in the body, but not the body. Keep the mind clean, the body clean and the heart dedicated. This is Yoga.*
>
> —H.H. SRI SWAMI SATCHIDANANDA

The Yoga for Health restorative program includes descriptions of how the poses specifically help the body recuperate from an acute or chronic disease, as in the case of patients diagnosed with diverse medical conditions affecting the immune and autoimmune, respiratory, neurologic, endocrine or musculoskeletal systems. I have found that having solid knowledge about how the different poses directly help the body recover is deeply helpful for my patients.

As mentioned in Part I, the Yoga for Health program model is predicated on the holistic, or "energetic," approach to healing the body—the same theory that forms the basis for acupuncture, acupressure, ayurveda and other "alternative" therapeutic modalities. By treating the internal systems, you're also treating the musculoskeletal system. And conversely, by treating the spine, muscles and joints, you contribute to the health of the internal organs, glands and nerves.

This book relies on a particular set of Hatha yoga poses, organized into a very specific, easy-to-do sequence. Once you begin practicing the Yoga for Health restorative program, the synergistic dynamic of the way the poses interact to support each physical system will begin to increase your strength and flexibility in surprising ways. The recuperative process of many patients who use the program is empirical. The Yoga for Health method is a hospital-proven formula that assists the body in its rehabilitation from a broad spectrum of acute and chronic diseases. If done daily—or at least three times a week—it can work for you.

CAVEAT: With the exception of variations, the two Yoga for Health programs (in Part I and Part II) include the same asansas in the same sequence. For therapeutic reasons, the asanas are organized in a specific sequence. They become progressively more difficult as the body becomes stronger and more flexible.

There are very subtle nerve centers situated along the spine that help regulate the natural energetic and organic functions of the physical (gross) nervous system. These subtle nerve centers, referred to by the ancient yoga masters as *Adhara Chakras,* correspond to the body's physical nerve centers (plexuses). Keeping these vital centers in harmonious balance is critical to the normal, healthy functioning of body and mind. When this balance is disrupted, the physical system begins to weaken and is more susceptible to various kinds of physical problems. The beginning Hatha yoga asanas in the Yoga for Health programs are set out in a particular sequence to maintain and restore the harmonious balance of the chakras, thereby producing the therapeutic effect necessary to both prevent and treat disease.

Beginning Level
CLASS TIME: 30 MINUTES

❀ ARDDHA PADMASANA (HALF LOTUS POSE) ❀

Sit with your legs stretched forward. Rest your right foot on your left thigh with the sole turned upward. Let your right knee touch the floor. Fold your left leg so that your left heel rests under your right thigh. Place your hands on your knees, palms up or down.

Clinical Benefits

This pose has been clinically noted to increase the output of blood from the heart, according to Dr. Sandra McLanahan, M.D., proving effective in the treatment of various forms of cardiovascular disease.

Beginning the Class

Sit in Half Lotus or assume a comfortable cross-legged position with your eyes closed. Use a wall for support if necessary. If unable to sit comfortably with your legs crossed, sit with them outstretched.

Bring your mental focus inward. Begin letting go of mental and physical distractions. Focusing on the flow of your breath can be helpful. Chant the "om" syllable three times to create a peaceful sensation in your nervous system and mind. Inhale. The "o" emanates from the abdomen and rises through the chest. The "m" consonant resonates in the head, stimulating the pineal gland in the center of the brain. The pineal gland releases the hormone melatonin, producing a centered, relaxed sensation in the mind and central nervous system.

The subtle sounds contained in mantras such as "om" are used by my patients at Cedars. UCLA Medical Center has a dedicated program for chanting, or "Kirtan," for cancer patients, and other physicians and healthcare practitioners such as cardiologist Dr. Mehmet Oz at New York Presbyterian Medical Center recommend the practice for their patients, as reported in *Time* magazine, October 6, 2003.

❧ NETHRA VYAYAMAM (EYE EXERCISES) ❧

For the eye exercises, use photo reference from Part I, on page 5.

In performing the eye exercises that follow, remember to do them slowly and with awareness. When your eyes are open, don't look at any particular object; simply focus on the natural movement of your eyes. Be careful not to strain. Center and close your eyes after each exercise.

1. Sitting in a cross-legged position, close your eyes and relax.
2. Open your eyes and move them from right to left four times.
3. Move your eyes up and down (from your forehead to your lap) four times.
4. Move your eyes in a clockwise rotation four times. Extend your gaze to the periphery.
5. Move your eyes in a counterclockwise rotation four times.
6. Bring your gaze back to the center and close your eyes.

Bring the palms of your hands together, brushing them back and forth until you create heat between them. Cup your palms over your eyes, allowing them to absorb the heat and energy from your hands, which helps to relax your eyes.

Clinical Benefits
These eye exercises help to relieve eye strain, tone the optic nerve and, in some cases, when practiced on a regular basis can improve vision.

SURYA NAMASKARA (SUN SALUTATION)

This is a series of twelve asanas (poses) done consecutively. One pose flows into the next in a smooth, dancelike fashion. There should be no strain involved. If during the course of doing this practice you experience any physical discomfort such as shortness of breath, a racing heart or nausea, or if you begin to perspire heavily, stop doing it and lie down in Savasana.

1. Stand with your legs together. Bring your palms together at your chest.
2. Lock your thumbs and stretch your arms straight out in front of you, then up, bending back slightly at the pelvis. Look up at your hands.
3. Bend forward and drop over your legs, keeping your knees straight. Bring your head toward your knees. Unlock your thumbs and relax your spine and arms.

4. Place the palms of your hands on the floor beside your feet (it's all right to bend your knees for comfort). Stretch your left leg back, placing the knee on the floor. Look up.
5. Stretch your right leg back to meet the left and raise your buttocks so you form a triangle, with your head between your arms. Look back at your feet. Gently stretch your heels toward the floor.
6. Lower your knees to the floor. Bring your chest and chin to the floor. Your chest should be positioned between your hands.
7. Press your pelvis to the floor and curl your spine and head up, keeping your elbows slightly bent. Do not push or strain.
8. Rise into the triangle pose again, looking back at your feet.
9. Lower your left knee to the floor, bring your right foot forward between your hands and look up.
10. Bring the left leg forward to meet the right and relax over your straightened legs, looking back at your knees.
11. Lock your thumbs together again, palms open. Stretch your arms up and back alongside your ears. Press your pelvis back slightly. Look back at your hands.
12. Return to an erect position, palms together at your chest.

Relax your arms alongside your body. Repeat twice.

CAVEAT: The Sun Salutation should not be performed by patients who are less than two months postoperative or otherwise clinically symptomatic without the consent of their physician or a certified yoga therapist.

Clinical Benefits

Stretches the entire body, increasing circulation into the heart, lungs and all the major organs, muscles and joints. It tones all the major muscle groups and promotes spinal alignment and flexibility, rejuvenating the nervous system. It stimulates the endocrine system, helping to support the immune function. It is beneficial in the prevention and treatment of arthritis by promoting the secretion of synovial fluid in the joints. For cardiac patients, it promotes cardiovascular circulation.

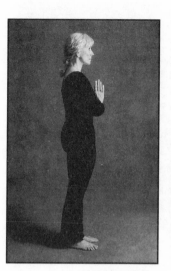
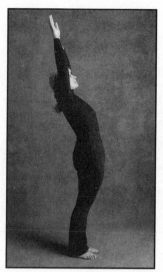
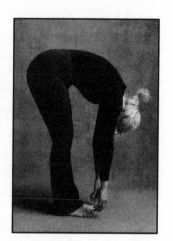

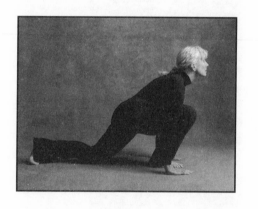
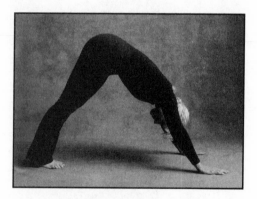

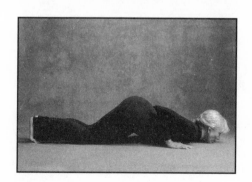
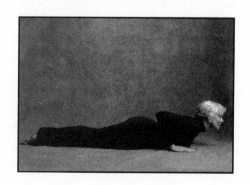

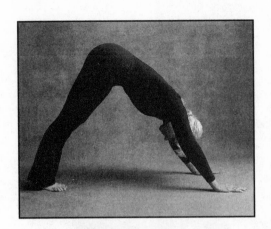

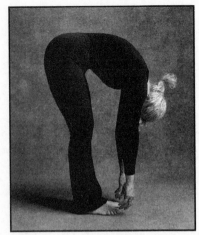

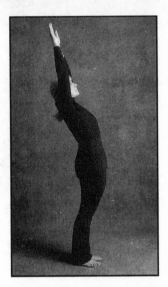

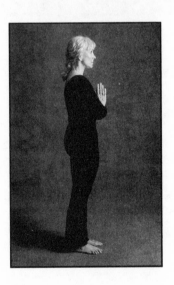

✿ SAVASANA (RELAXATION POSE) ✿

Lie on your back with your arms and legs extended and your palms up. Close your eyes. Your legs should be about eighteen inches apart.

This pose is done between asanas to allow the body to rest completely and experience the benefit of the pose just performed. For people with back discomfort or who have been diagnosed with a back condition, use a small pillow or place a rolled towel under the knees to help relieve pressure from the dorsal (mid) spine. A support can also be used under the neck for comfort, if necessary.

BHUJANGASANA (COBRA POSE)

To prepare, lie on your stomach in *Savasana* (Relaxation Pose), your arms alongside your body and your cheek to one side. Your legs should be about seventeen inches apart. Bring your forehead to the floor. Place your palms on the floor, below your shoulders, elbows raised and close to the trunk of your body. Relax all your muscles completely. Bring your legs close together with your toes pointed.

Now slowly raise your head and bend your neck back as far as possible. Slowly raise your chest, bending your vertebrae backward one by one. Keep your elbows bent. Inhale while rising, breathe normally in the pose and exhale coming down. Hold for ten seconds. Repeat twice or according to your strength and ability.

CAVEAT: This asana is contraindicated (not recommended) for postoperative patients (i.e., following bypass surgery) who have sutures in their chest, and should not be performed until the thoracic area has completely healed and the patient can lie comfortably on his or her stomach. Consult with your physician or yoga therapist before attempting this pose.

Clinical Benefits

Stimulates the thyroid gland at the base of throat, helping to stabilize metabolism and lower blood cholesterol, which helps in the treatment of cardiovascular disease and other conditions. The back muscles are strengthened. The spine becomes more supple and the chest expands, promoting oxygen and circulation into the lungs and heart, which is helpful in the treatment of asthma. The cranial nerves at the base of the skull are stimulated, promoting activity and tone and helping to both prevent and treat headaches and migraines. The thymus gland in the center of the chest is stimulated, helping to strengthen the immune function. This pose also eases backache caused by strain, and constipation and flatulence. Vertabrae displaced in the spine are subtly adjusted. In women, the ovaries and uterus are toned by increased circulation, helping to alleviate various utero-ovarian complaints.

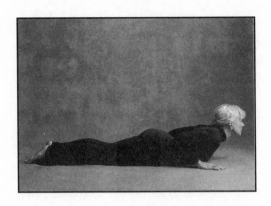

❁ ARDDHASALABASANA (HALF LOCUST POSE) ❁

Lie facedown with your chin on the floor. Tuck your arms beneath your body, palms up, beneath your thighs. Do not bend your elbows. Keep your toes pointed. Raise your right leg without bending the knee. Allow all your weight to rest on your chest and arms. Slowly lower the leg. Relax. Do the same with the left leg. Turn your head to the side and rest. Keep your arms in place and return your chin to the floor. Repeat. Perform twice with each leg.

Clinical Benefits

The back, pelvis and abdomen are toned and strengthened, helping in the treatment of lower-back weakness, tightness and spasm. The disk space between the spinal vertebrae is stretched, helping to promote spinal alignment. The sympathetic nervous system (the portion of the nervous system devoted to arousal for fight or flight, located in the mid back) is balanced, helping in the treatment of heart disease. Pressure increases in the heart and lungs, helping in their elasticity and lymph drainage. This pose increases circulation and massages the prostate or the uterus and ovaries, helpful in the treatment of prostate or uterine disease.

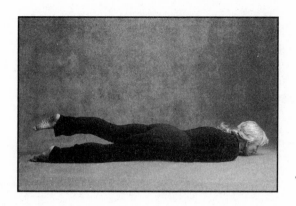

SAVASANA

JANUSIRASANA (HEAD-TO-KNEE POSE)

Postoperative patients should be careful in performing this pose. Avoid doing it if it aggravates the chest or abdominal area.

Sit on the floor with your legs outstretched. Bring your left heel into the groin area with the sole of your left foot resting against your right inner thigh. Lock your thumbs and raise your arms overhead, stretching your spine up.

Look up at your hands, keep your head aligned between your arms and bend forward over your extended leg. Bring your face to your knee, keeping your leg straight. Relax into the pose. Avoid straining.

Repeat the pose, bending over your left leg. Perform once with each leg. Hold for a maximum of ten seconds.

Clinical Benefits

Helps to relieve constipation. Stimulates the vagus nerve, toning the parasympathetic nervous system and increasing blood flow to the heart. Helps in the treatment of heart disease. Reduces plaque in the coronary arteries and lowers cholesterol. Because of the improved circulation and gentle massaging of the lower bowel in practicing this pose, the medical benefits include prevention and treatment of constipation and hemorrhoids. The additional stimulation to the parasympathetic nervous system also contributes to improved bowel action and relief of constipation.

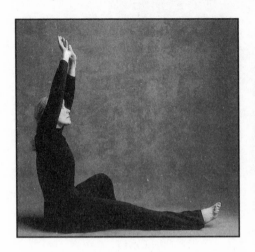 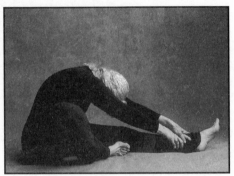

SAVASANA

✺ JANISHURSASANA (SUPPORTED) ✺

For those limited in flexibility, who are unable to sit on the floor in an unsupported position, the following modifications are an option:

1. Wall support. Lean against the wall, making sure the base of the spine is against the flat surface. Bring the left heel into the groin area with the right leg extended. Lock the thumbs and stretch your arms upward toward the ceiling. Look up at your hands, inhale and on the exhalation bend forward over the extended leg. Hold for ten seconds or according to your capacity.

2. Chair pose: Sit in a straight-back chair. Lock the thumbs and raise your arms overhead. Inhale and on the exhalation lean forward over the right leg, grasping the leg where it's comfortable. It's all right to bend the knee if necessary. Relax your face and neck toward the leg. Breathe comfortably in the pose. Hold for ten seconds or according to comfort. To come out of the pose, lock the thumbs and raise the arms overhead, then relax the arms in the lap. Or just sit up comfortably.

SAVASANA

✾ PASCHIMOTHANASANA (FULL FORWARD BEND) ✾

Lie on your back. Stretch your arms over your head, if you can do so comfortably, and lock your thumbs. Slowly raise your arms, head and chest, sitting up into an upright position. If you find this too difficult, just sit up comfortably. Then stretch your arms over your head and lock the thumbs.

Slowly bend forward over your legs as far as you can comfortably go. Grasp your legs wherever you can reach comfortably—your ankles, calves or thighs. Relax your face into your knees if you are able to. Otherwise, relax your head to your chest. Relax in this position, breathing normally, for ten seconds. Keep the legs straight, or if necessary bend them for your comfort.

To come out of this pose, lock your thumbs and stretch out over your legs, then rise into an upright position. Bring your hands to your lap and lie back comfortably in a supine position.

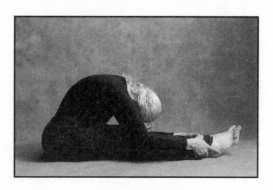

✾ PASCHIMOTHANASANA (SUPPORTED) ✾

Wall: Sit against the wall and as you inhale, bend forward over the extended legs. Exhale and grasp the knees, calves or ankles, or wherever you can reach comfortably. Relax the neck and shoulders, bringing your face and head forward toward the legs. Breathe normally in the pose. Hold for ten seconds or according to your capacity. To come out of the pose, lock your thumbs and stretch your arms out over the extended legs and rise slowly. Or just sit up comfortably.

Chair: Sit in a comfortable chair. Extend your legs in front of you and bend forward, grasping the knees, calves or ankles, or wherever you can reach comfortably. Bring your face and head toward the legs. Breathe normally in the pose. Hold for ten seconds or according to your own capacity. To come out of the pose, gently rise to a seated position in your chair and relax.

Clinical Benefits

Stimulates, massages and relaxes the pelvic floor. In particular it stretches the sacroiliac junction, helpful in the treatment of lower backache as well as sciatica (the painful pinching of the root to the sciatic nerve that can manifest as pain in one or both buttocks or down one or both legs).

CAVEAT: Do not practice this pose if you have a disease of the abdominal viscera, or enlargement of the liver or spleen.

SAVASANA

SARVANGASANA (SHOULDERSTAND): STANDARD VERSION

Adjust your clothing to loosen any restrictions in movement. Lie on your back with your feet together and your arms alongside your body, palms down. Inhale, straighten your legs and lift them over your head in a horizontal position. (If necessary, bend your knees in order to raise them over your head.) Then straighten your legs into a vertical position, keeping them together. Bring your palms to your lower back for support. Begin breathing normally. Keep the chin tucked into your chest. Hold for one to three minutes, according to your capacity. You can gradually build to five minutes as you become stronger.

To come out of the pose, lower your legs over your head, parallel to the floor.

Bring the arms to the floor for support. Slowly roll the spine to the floor, keeping the legs straight if you can. Otherwise, bend the knees as you come down. Continue breathing normally.

The mental focus in this pose is the base of the throat. Do not sneeze, cough or yawn while in the pose. Come out of the pose immediately if you experience nausea, dizziness, shortness of breath, perspiration or fullness or pressure in the neck or head. If you need to cough, swallow or sneeze, come out of the pose to avoid choking.

Clinical Benefits

Regulates the thyroid gland and stabilizes the metabolism; helpful in the treatment of overactive and underactive thyroid conditions. Stimulates the baroreceptors in the neck, lowering blood pressure and pulse rate and thereby helpful in the treatment of heart disease such as cardiomyopathy and coronary artery disease.

This pose also balances the sympathetic and parasympathetic nervous systems, further helping to support the cardiovascular system. It stimulates the pineal and pituitary glands in the center of the brain, thereby balancing the sympathetic and parasympathetic nervous systems and further helping in the treatment of heart disease such as cardiomyopathy and coronary artery disease. Because of the increased blood and lymph drainage toward the upper body, when you stand up, the flow of these fluids into your legs and lower organs provides therapy for varicose veins and hemorrhoids—conditions that result from the excessive pressure of gravity on the valves in the veins.

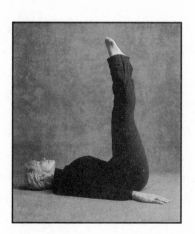
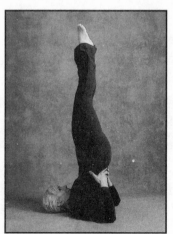

SARVANGASANA (SHOULDERSTAND): MODIFIED VERSION

(a) Lie on your back and elevate your legs to a 90-degree angle. Hold for one to three minutes according to your capacity.

(b) Lie on your back with your legs elevated on a chair. Hold this position for three minutes, or come out of the pose sooner if you become uncomfortable or experience symptomatology such as pressure or the feeling of fullness in the head or neck, shortness of breath, a racing heart, nausea, dizziness or perspiration.

(c) Lie on your back with your legs elevated on a wall.

Use these modifications if you have severe high blood pressure, back pain, neck or shoulder injuries or other physiological limitations. Postoperative patients should use either of these modifications for two months before attempting to do the standard version.

SAVASANA

MATSYASANA (FISH POSE)

Lie flat on the floor with your palms pressed against the sides of your thighs. Shift your bodyweight to your elbows and raise your head and trunk. Arch your chest and lower the crown of your head to the floor, creating a "bridge" between your buttocks and head. Expand your chest as much as possible and place a smile on your lips to break up tension in your jaw.

To come out of the pose, place your bodyweight on your elbows again and raise your head gently. Then slowly roll your spine to the floor. Deep breathing through your nose enhances the benefit of the practice. Do not hold your breath. Hold for approximately five seconds, increasing the time as you become more proficient.

CAVEAT: Do not swallow while doing this pose. If you feel like coughing or sneezing, come out of the pose before doing so. Do not do this posture if you have a headache or fever, or if you suffer from any disturbance in the cranial organs.

Clinical Benefits

Increases circulation to the lungs. As reported in the *Journal of the American Medical Association* (*JAMA*), this pose has been clinically recognized to be effective in treating asthma and bronchial conditions. By extending the cervical and thoracic spine backward, the neck and upper back and chest muscles are stretched and stimulated, increasing flexibility and circulation to them. Because it improves circulation to the thyroid, this pose helps the thyroid gland regulate itself so it is neither over- nor underactive, thereby stabilizing metabolism. It also increases blood flow to the cardiovascular system, helping in the treatment of heart disease.

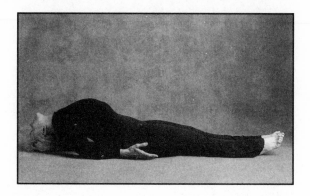

SAVASANA

PAVANAMUKTASANA (WIND ELIMINATION)

Lie flat on your back. Raise both legs to your chest while drawing in a deep breath through your nose. Hold the breath. Raise your head and bring it to your knees. Exhale slowly, release your legs and lie back on the floor with your arms and legs extended.

CLINICAL NOTE: Postoperative cardiac patients should not do this pose until the chest area is no longer irritated or symptomatic.

Clinical Benefits
Relieves strain and tightness in the lower back. It massages the abdominal organs and digestive tract, increasing circulation and pushing the contents of the bowel along, thus helping to relieve constipation. Any accumulated gas is expelled, relieving the pressure of flatulence.

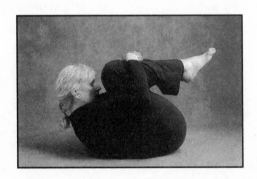

SAVASANA

❀ ARDDHAMATSYANDRASANA (HALF SPINAL TWIST) ❀

Sit on the floor and bring your knees to your chest. Extend your right leg straight up. Cross your right foot over your left knee, placing the sole of your right foot flat on the floor. Sitting up straight, bring your right knee close to your chest. Now extend your arms in front of you, locking your thumbs and twisting to the right. Unlock your thumbs and place your right hand on the floor behind you, close to your body, with your fingers pointing away from you. Place your left arm between your trunk and your right knee (i.e., on the outside of your right knee) and press your knee to the right. You can also wrap your left arm around your right knee, bringing it close to your chest. Slowly twist your head and trunk to the right and look over your right shoulder. Hold for five seconds to begin with, gradually increasing to ten seconds as you progress. Then slowly unwind, coming back to center. Bring both knees to your chest, then repeat the pose with your left leg.

CLINICAL NOTE: Postoperative cardiac patients with chest sutures should not do this pose until the chest area is no longer irritated or symptomatic.

Clinical Benefits

Increases circulation to the liver, spleen, kidneys, gallbladder and adrenal glands. The twisting motion increases pressure and circulation to the abdominal cavity and organs, helping to relieve constipation. It tones the sympathetic nerves and ganglia (nerve bundles) in the mid and lower back, reducing stress levels and helping in the treatment of obesity. It also strengthens the deep (lower) and superficial (upper and middle) muscles of the back, which hold up the spine and keep the vertebrae in place.

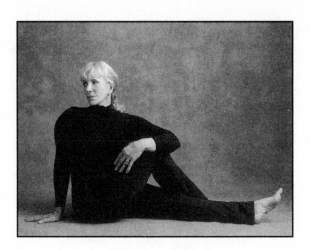

❀ YOGA MUDRA (YOGIC SEAL) ❀

Sit on the floor in a comfortable cross-legged position. Place your hands behind your back and grasp your right wrist with your left hand. Inhale, slowly bend forward and touch the floor with your forehead first and then, gradually, your chin. If you have only a limited range of motion, just relax forward as far as you can and relax your chin to your chest. The focus is the center of your forehead. On the exhalation, stretch your chin out and slowly rise.

Clinical Benefits
Gently massages the digestive tract, helping move food along and thereby preventing constipation. By increasing circulation to the pancreas, it helps improve this gland's function, thus assisting in the prevention and treatment of obesity. The sympathetic nerves—the portion of the nervous system located in the mid back, consisting of nerve fibers and ganglia (masses of nerve cell bodies located along the spinal column)—are stimulated, as are the parasympathetic nerves in the lower back. This activity helps relax the body and center the mind. It also strengthens both the deep *erector spinae* muscles that support the lumbar spine and the superficial *latissimus dorsi* muscles of the mid back.

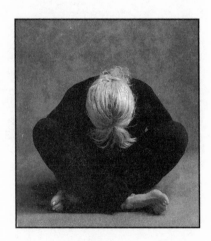

❧ YOGA NIDRA (DEEP RELAXATION) ❧

Lie on your back in a comfortable supine position with your arms and legs extended. The legs should be about a foot and a half apart, the arms a few inches away from the body. Close your eyes and, breathing through your nose, begin relaxing into the position.

Bring your awareness to your right leg and foot. Begin tensing the leg. Lift it off the floor a few inches. Tense a little more, then let it gently drop. Roll it from side to side and just forget about it. Repeat with the left leg.

Now inhale and tense your pelvis and buttocks. Squeeze the tension out. Most of us hold a lot of stress in this area, which can lead to disorders in the reproductive system as well as in the pelvis and hips. Now inhale and fill your stomach with air. Hold for a few moments, then release through your mouth. Just let it gush out. Inhale again, filling your stomach with air. Then bring it into your chest. Hold it. Open your mouth and let it gush out. Experience the warm sensation of the release.

Bring your awareness to your right hand and arm. Inhale, close your hand into a gentle fist and begin tensing tightly all the way to your shoulder. Then release. Repeat with your left hand and arm.

Inhale and raise your shoulders to your ears. Hold for a moment. Then release. Turn your head from side to side slowly. Then center and relax. Bring your awareness to your face. Open your mouth and drop your jaw. Move it from side to side. Then center and relax. Now tense your face into a tight prune face. And release. Open your mouth wide and extend your tongue as far as you can. And then relax. Your body should be completely relaxed and free of tension at this point.

To begin the second phase of the practice, without moving, bring your mental awareness to your feet. Begin mentally relaxing your feet. Now bring your mental awareness up your entire body, relaxing each part until you reach your head. Once your body is free of all stress, bring your mental awareness to your breath. Begin observing the flow of your breath. Just watch the gentle inhalation and exhalation. You'll notice that your breath becomes increasingly subtle. It might seem like you're not breathing at all. Don't worry. You are.

Just watch yourself becoming more and more relaxed as your breath becomes more "invisible" and subtle. I have known some clients to become afraid at this point, when the breath is very still. It's not uncommon. If you can, just keep relaxing through it. The breath is just deepening. You're breathing on a subtler level that is much more therapeutic than the breathing we're accustomed to.

At this point, when your breath is quite still, bring your awareness to your mind. Begin watching your mind. Observe your thoughts as they enter and leave your mind. You most likely will find that your mind begins to fill with random thoughts at this point, particularly if you are new to this practice. It's a common experience. The important thing is not to push the thoughts away. Don't force anything. Just continue watching the phenomenon as though you're watching a film. After doing this practice a few times you will find that eventually your mind will begin to relax and let go of the thoughts. Then you'll begin to experience a very relaxed, blissful quality within yourself. This is where the healing takes place—in this very subtle and peaceful energy within yourself.

As you come out of your relaxation, slowly bring your awareness back to your breath and let it gradually deepen. Imagine that you're breathing all the way into your feet. Let your awareness rise through your body, waking up all the parts until you reach your head. Then begin gently moving all parts of your body. Observe the relaxed and easeful quality within them.

You can now slowly rise and begin preparation for the *pranayama* (breathing practices).

For optimal benefit in a formal class it's customary for this silent relaxation part of the practice to last for fifteen minutes. You can customize the time to accommodate your schedule when doing it on your own. There is an audiotape of the yoga nidra practice recorded by Swami Satchidananda that I use with my cardiac patients at Cedars-Sinai Medical Center. Many of my private clients have told me that they enjoy this tape and that it helps them in their practice. See Resources (page 264) for more details.

Clinical Benefits

Reduces stress in the muscles, organs and nervous system. Allows the heart to rest deeply, thereby stabilizing blood pressure and promoting a profound sense of well-being throughout the entire system. For this reason, this practice is highly recommended for treatment of cardiovascular disease as well as immune and endocrine-related conditions.

Pranayama (Breathing Practices)

CLINICAL NOTE: For patients with cardiac, immune or endocrine-related conditions, the pranayama practices should be done at least three times a day.

DEERGA SWASAM (DEEP BREATHING)

Exhale completely through your nose. Place your right hand on your chest and your left hand on your abdomen. Inhale and fill your abdominal area with air. As you do this, your left hand will begin to rise but your right hand will not. After filling your abdomen with air, keep inhaling and allow more air to fill your lower chest. This will cause your right hand to rise. Your rib cage will expand as you inhale. Continue inhaling, bringing the air higher into your chest to the collarbone, causing it to rise.

On the exhalation, slowly expel the air, deflating the upper chest, rib cage and abdomen. Bring the abdomen toward the spine. Do this for at least one minute.

NADDI SUDDHI (ALTERNATE NOSTRIL BREATHING)

Close your right hand into a loose, comfortable fist. Extend your thumb and last two fingers. You can also use your thumb and forefinger if it's easier. Close the right nostril with your right thumb. Quietly expel the air out of your left nostril. Inhale through your left nostril and close it with your last two fingers and exhale through your right nostril.

Continue doing this practice, alternating breath between nostrils. Once you're comfortable with the coordination, establish a 1:2 ratio between the inhalation and exhalation. The exhalation should be twice as long as the inhalation (i.e., inhale "one om, two om," exhale "one om, two om, three om, four om").

Do this for at least one minute in the beginning. On the final exhalation, exhale through your right nostril. Let the breath return to normal. Sit and quietly observe the effects of the breathing practice on your system.

MEDICAL MODELS

If you think about disaster, brood about death, you hasten your disease. Think positively and masterfully and with confidence and faith. Your life will become more secure, more fraught with action, richer in achievement and experience.

—Swami Sivananda, Sat Guru, Physician

The doctor of the future will give no medicine but will interest his patients in the care of the human frame and diet and in the cause and prevention of disease.

—Thomas Edison, Scientist, Inventor

First the doctor gave me the good news. I was going to have a disease named after me.

—Steve Martin, Actor

The following medical models present a comprehensive clinical perspective on the body's primary physical systems and their related diseases and how yoga can be specifically relevant, as an adjunct therapy, in their rehabilitation. Each dedicated section includes a recommendation for specific postures for each physical system and its related conditions.

Again, as with acupuncture and other forms of what is referred to as "energetic" and "holistic" medicine, yoga places an emphasis on generally strengthening and rebalancing the whole of a particular body system in the treatment of disease. For example, in treating colon cancer, the various organs of the immune system are strengthened, in addition to the affected organ itself, in order to achieve a comprehensive effect.

COMMON AILMENTS

There is nothing new under the sun.

—ECCLESIASTES 1:9

Natural forces within us are the true healers of disease.

—HIPPPOCRATES

The best doctors in the world are Doctor Diet, Doctor Quiet,
and Doctor Merryman.

—JONATHAN SWIFT

Which Yoga for Health program to use in conjunction with the recommended asanas in this Common Ailments section depends on your general physical health and level of flexibility. For those practitioners and patients who are not postoperative and have a full range of motion, the Yoga for Health Practice Set I (pages 3–30) is recommended. Those practitioners and patients who are six months or fewer postoperative or have physical limitations should use Practice Set II (pages 89–112).

Insomnia

How often do you toss and turn restlessly in bed, unable to fall asleep? You lie there, counting the minutes, waiting and hoping for the adrenaline rush to shift and drowsiness to take over. Knowing you're going to have to be up at 6 A.M., rested, with functioning brain cells, focused, articulate and ready to choreograph the day for a family of five, perform brain surgery, anchor the early morning news, take that final exam, make that all-important business pitch, strategize your boss's stock portfolio, drive the Indy 500 or take that long shot that's going to define the rest of your professional life. All you want is a good night's sleep. You do mental math. You try sleep affirmations. You listen to whale sounds. You turn on C-SPAN, hoping to be anesthetized. Nothing works.

> *The human body is a temple. Keep it strong and supple. To purify the body practice the disciplines of Hatha yoga and take care of your diet.*
>
> —H.H. Sri Swami Satchidananda

Desperately, you consider running out to the all-night pharmacy and knocking yourself out with the soothing sleeping aids so seductively promoted on late-night TV. But then the invisible announcer hyperkinetically rattles off the list of potentially harmful and life-threatening side effects: dizziness, dry mouth, tongue-swelling and the inability to talk, daytime drowsiness, rapid heart palpitations, anxiety, panic attacks, apathy, blurred vision with risk of blindness, dyslexia, impaired judgment, spatial disorientation, bleeding ulcers with associated gum discharge, thinning hair, incontinence, sexual dysfunction, lowered sperm count in men, debilitating memory loss, manic depression leading to psychosis, drug addiction, and constipation leading to acute bowel disease, which in some cases can be fatal. I don't know. Is it really worth a night's sleep?

In the United States alone, statistics show that approximately one-third of all adults suffer from some type of sleep disorder. The Mayo Clinic states that insomnia is the most common of these disorders. It is defined as the inability to fall asleep after lying in bed for thirty minutes, or the inabililty to sustain sleep for more than a few hours without waking. Some of the common clinical factors that can cause insomnia are stress, a poor diet and things that interfere with the body's normal sleep cycles, such as shift work and jet lag.

According to Dr. Carrie Angus, medical director of the Himalayan Institute for Yoga Science and Philosophy, our bodies are designed for sleep to come effortlessly. When it doesn't, it's because we're holding on to the day's stresses and, at the same time, projecting tomorrow's.

While it requires a little more discipline and planning on your part than simply popping a pill, there is a less risky solution. Sat Bir Singh Khalsa, S.D., of Brigham and Women's Hospital, Harvard Medical School, verifies that certain Hatha yoga and relaxation techniques are effective for specific sleep disorders. Hatha yoga and meditation relieve stress from the endocrine and nervous systems, helping the body reregulate itself, thereby inducing the mind and body to let go and slip gently into a deep, restful sleep. Doing the adjunct practices (outlined below) once a day, along with the Yoga for Health Practice Set I or II at least once a week, can be helpful in allowing you to regulate your body into a healthy sleep pattern.

In addition to the Hatha yoga practices I recommend, I strongly advise you to adopt a diet that is more conducive to a restful sleep and make suitable changes in your sleeping environment. Adjusting your dietary habits requires limiting your intake of stimulants such as caffeine, alcohol and spicy foods, and avoiding them altogether at night. Keeping your environment free from external stressors will allow your body and mind to relax more comfortably.

Recommended Asanas

JANUSIRASANA (HEAD-TO-KNEE POSE)

Stimulates the parasympathetic nervous system, helping in the relaxation response.

SARVANGASANA (SHOULDERSTAND)

Induces relaxation throughout the body by stimulating the pineal gland, releasing the hormone melatonin into the nervous system.

MATSYASANA (FISH POSE)

Stimulates the thyroid gland, helping to regulate the metabolism.

✾ YOGA NIDRA (DEEP RELAXATION) ✾

(To be done at bedtime)

Releases stress from the system, allowing the heart to rest more deeply.

✾ NADDI SUDDHI (ALTERNATE NOSTRIL BREATHING) ✾

(To be done at least once during the day and at bedtime)

Balances the sympathetic and parasympathetic nervous systems.

The Common Cold

The common cold may be caused by a variety of viruses and is characterized by a runny nose, sneezing and a sore throat. Our ability to fight viruses depends on the strength of our immune system. Our immune system consists of white blood cells that circulate in the blood and the organs of the thymus (located in the chest above the heart) and the spleen (located in the right upper abdomen). In addition, bone marrow acts to manufacture white blood cells.

Each patient carries his own doctor inside him. We are at our best when we give the doctor who resides within each patient a chance to go to work.

—ALBERT SCHWEITZER, M.D.

Immunity is impacted by both physical and mental factors. Because the sequences of yoga stretches enhance circulation, they can help white blood cells meet their targets, preventing infection. In addition, as the body and mind relax via the Yoga for Health program, the immune system becomes more efficient in producing adequate amounts of white blood cells. If your energy is focused on dealing with stress (in fight-or-flight mode), fewer white blood cells will be available for effective work. Because of this, stress has been found to affect your likelihood of developing a cold. For example, students catch more colds at exam time. Actors in one study were found to have less activity in their immune system even just by thinking negative thoughts.

The hormone cortisol may be the trigger. Stress elevates cortisol levels, and cortisol lowers white blood cell function. Regular yoga practice—even just one class a week—has been found to lower cortisol levels.

If, despite yoga practice, you experience the first symptoms of a cold, you can help stop it in its tracks by doing the Shoulderstand to draw blood to your head and throat. This brings more white blood cells to the areas where they're needed and helps relieve sinus congestion.

> *I finally realized that being grateful to my body meant beginning to give more love to myself.*
>
> —Oprah Winfrey

In addition, deep relaxation followed by pranayama can help the body relax enough to focus its energies on fighting the infection. It also allows you to rest more deeply during your recovery.

Recommended Asanas

SARVANGASANA (SHOULDERSTAND)

Brings blood to the head and throat, relieving sinus congestion. Reduces stress, helping to strengthen the immune function.

MATSYASANA (FISH POSE)

Opens up the throat and lungs, increasing circulation and thereby helping to break up congestion.

YOGA NIDRA (DEEP RELAXATION)

Allows the heart to rest deeply. Reduces stress, helping to strengthen the immune system.

Flu

Influenza is caused by various strains of viruses. In contrast to the common cold, viruses cause a more systemic (whole-body) illness characterized by aches and

pains, often accompanied by fever. Susceptibility to infection by influenza depends on the competence of the body's immune system. The regular practice of yoga can help prevent influenza virus infections.

Should you develop the flu, focus mainly on deep relaxation, pranayama and visualization. They help relieve aching limbs and allow your system to focus on fighting off the virus.

Recommended Asanas

YOGA NIDRA (DEEP RELAXATION)

Reduces stress in the entire system, helping to strengthen the immune functions.

NADDI SUDDHI (ALTERNATE NOSTRIL BREATHING)

Balances the sympathetic (active) and parasympathetic (relaxation response) nervous systems, thereby reducing stress.

VISUALIZATION

Visualize your system being completely filled with healing, restorative energy. Imagine your white blood cells—your body's tactical defense force—mobilized and strategically fighting off the virus infection, helping to restore your body's immunity.

PMS: Premenstrual Syndrome

According to the Mayo Clinic, as many as 75 percent of women in the United States suffer from PMS, or premenstrual syndrome. While the demographic for this condition is twenty-to-thirty-year-olds, it is not necessarily limited to this age group.

Common symptoms of PMS include bloating, tender breasts, irritability and mood swings, depression and general malaise. Not all women are aware of the transient personality aberrations affecting them until they walk into a room and it clears, or their behavior is brought to their attention by a spouse, family member, business associate, coworker or some other daring individual who, at great personal risk, alludes to it being "your time of month." You feel like you weigh 500 pounds. Your body, while portable, has become a piece of heavy equipment.

As many as half of all women in the United States may experience this condition. Although the exact mechanism is unclear, emotional stress appears to play a significant role in the hormonal imbalance believed to cause this problem.

Both Yoga for Health programs (Set I and II) may alleviate these hormonal irregularities because they reduce stress and allow the muscles to relax deeply. When muscles are less tense they require less blood, so more is available for the body's repair mechanisms. A vegetarian diet has also been shown to be associated with a decreased rate of PMS due to a shift in estrogen levels in relation to progesterone.

Recommended Asanas

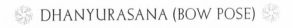

DHANYURASANA (BOW POSE)

Increases circulation to the nerve plexes in the lower back (parasympathetic nervous system), helping to relax the nervous system. Promotes circulation in the ovaries and uterus. Increases circulation in the digestive system (colon and small intestine), helping to relieve constipation.

JANUSIRASANA (HEAD-TO-KNEE POSE)

Stimulates the parasympathetic nervous system. Increases circulation to the digestive system, uterus and ovaries.

PASCHIMOTHANASANA (FULL FORWARD BEND)

Stretches out the lower back, helping to relieve tension in the lumbar paraspinals (musculature). Applies gentle pressure to the abdominal muscles, increasing circulation in the colon and small intestine. Tones the parasympathetic nerves.

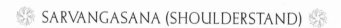

SARVANGASANA (SHOULDERSTAND)

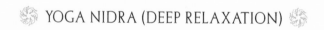

YOGA NIDRA (DEEP RELAXATION)

Both of these practices are especially helpful in the treatment of PMS by balancing the endocrine (hormonal) system and stimulating the pineal, thymus and thyroid glands. They increase circulation into all the major organs.

MATSYASANA (FISH POSE)

Stimulates the thyroid gland in the base of the throat, helping to regulate metabolism. Stimulates the pineal gland in the center of the brain, releasing melatonin, which brings a relaxed response to the nervous system.

NADDI SUDDHI (ALTERNATE NOSTRIL BREATHING)

Balances the sympathetic (active) nervous system with the parasympathetic (relaxation) nervous system, helping to restore balance to the mind, glands and organs.

Menstrual Cramps

Menstrual cramps may be precipitated by hormonal imbalance and stress. The relaxing effect of yoga poses can make a significant impact on both preventing and relieving this muscle cramping. Wind Elimination, the Bow Pose, Head-to-Knee Pose, Full Forward Bend and Shoulderstand may be especially helpful in preventing these symptoms. Cramping can also be caused by impeded circulation in the ovaries and uterus, stress in the kidneys and sluggish bowels. If cramps develop, deep relaxation and alternate nostril breathing are the best remedies.

> *I was going to have cosmetic surgery until I noticed that the doctor's office was full of portraits by Picasso.*
>
> —RITA RUDNER

Recommended Asanas

PAVANAMUKTASANA (WIND ELIMINATION)

Relieves gas and constipation.

🏵 DHANYURASANA (BOW POSE) 🏵

Relieves lower-back strain and increases circulation in the uterus and ovaries. A vegetarian diet has also been shown to alleviate menstrual cramps.

Menopause

Menopause is a natural biological process that occurs in women. According to the Mayo Clinic, menopause is not an isolated event but a slow transition in the hormonal system. It can begin when a woman is in her thirties or forties, or not until her sixties. Further reports by the Mayo Clinic assert that menopause does not signal the end of youth or vitality, or sexual activity, which can continue into the later years, even well into the eighties.

> *You're never too old to become younger.*
> —MAE WEST

A woman's lifestyle, including diet, stress levels and mental attitude, can significantly affect the symptoms of hot flashes, depression and mood swings caused by hormonal imbalances. For example, menopause symptoms are reported to be significantly higher among women in the United States than those in Asian and European countries due to stress.

The increased circulation achieved by yoga practice can help keep tissues healthy at menopause. Hormonal imbalances may be more easily corrected when the body is regularly relaxed.

Recommended Asanas

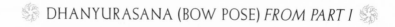

🏵 DHANYURASANA (BOW POSE) *FROM PART I* 🏵

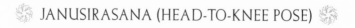

🏵 JANUSIRASANA (HEAD-TO-KNEE POSE) 🏵

SARVANGASANA (SHOULDERSTAND):
SUPPORTED OR UNSUPPORTED

YOGA NIDRA (DEEP RELAXATION)

NADDI SUDDHI (ALTERNATE NOSTRIL BREATHING)

A vegetarian diet acts to prevent hot flashes and other menopausal symptoms because it is high in phytoestrogens from plants.

Constipation

The United States is one of the most constipated countries in the world. This is mainly due to inadequate fiber in the diet. We should eat at least 30 to 40 grams of fiber per day, whereas on average Americans consume only 5 grams. Switching to a vegetarian diet is the most important first step in the prevention and treatment of constipation.

The gentle massaging action of the yoga postures in the digestive tract, which moves the food along, can significantly help in the prevention and treatment of constipation.

> *We are fond of one another because our ailments are the same.*
>
> —JONATHAN SWIFT

Recommended Asanas

SURYA NAMASKARA (SUN SALUTATION)

Circulates blood and lymph throughout the entire system, helping to energize the digestive function.

✸ JANUSIRASANA (HEAD-TO-KNEE POSE) ✸

Applies gentle pressure to the abdominal area, helping to move food through.

✸ SARVANGASANA (SHOULDERSTAND) ✸

Draws blood into the abdominal plexus, helping to promote digestion.

✸ ARDDHAMATSYANDRASANA (HALF SPINAL TWIST) ✸

The twisting motion increases circulation into the colon and small intestine, increasing blood flow and helping to move food along.

✸ PAVANAMUKTASANA (WIND ELIMINATION) ✸

Applies additional pressure to the abdomen, stimulating the colon and small intestine. Helps to move food through the digestive tract.

✸ KAPALA BATHI (SKULL SHINING) ✸

Increases energy in the colon and small intestine, helping to process food.

Prostate Gland Disease

Increased fat in the diet is felt to be a trigger for prostate disease. The excess fat may interfere directly with circulation or shift hormone balances to encourage tumor formation and growth.

By assisting in the maintenance of calm awareness, yoga practices may help practitioners regulate their dietary fat intake. In addition, by placing the body in the various postures of yoga, improved circulation and nutrient delivery may help the body in its self-regulatory activity for maintaining optimum cell health. This may help prevent prostate cancer and other conditions related to the prostate gland.

Once a tumor has developed, yoga practice can reduce stress during this difficult time. It also helps support the immune function in its ability to fight the disease.

> As to diseases make a habit of two things—to help, or at least, to do no harm.
>
> —HIPPPOCRATES, *EPIDEMICS*

Recommended Asanas

JANUSHIRSASANA (HEAD-TO-KNEE POSE)

The gentle pressure applied by the heel to the genitalia helps to stimulate circulation into the organs and prostate gland. Induces parasympathetic nervous system response, helping to promote relaxation, thereby enhancing immune function.

SARVANGASANA (SHOULDERSTAND)

(To be done either supported or unsupported)

Regulates the thyroid gland and stabilizes the metabolism; helpful in the treatment of overactive or underactive thyroid conditions. Stimulates the baroreceptors in the neck, lowering blood pressure and pulse rate. Stimulates the pineal and pituitary glands in the center of the brain, thereby balancing the sympathetic and parasympathetic nervous systems and futher helping in the treatment of immune-related disorders such as cancer, chronic fatigue, AIDS and the flu (see Common Ailments, page 115).

> *Hard work never killed anybody, but why take a chance?*
>
> —EDGAR BERGEN (CHARLIE MCCARTHY)

MATSYASANA (FISH POSE)

Because this pose improves circulation to the thyroid, it helps this gland regulate itself so that it is neither over- nor underactive, thereby stabilizing metabolism. It increases blood flow into the cardiovascular system, helping support various glands and organs such as the thymus gland (in the chest above the heart) and spleen (in the right upper abdomen), helping the white blood cells that make up the immune system circulate and target infection.

Headaches and Migraines

Headaches are the most common health problem in the United States. Simple tension and eye strain are the usual cause. Poses to emphasize in conjunction with the Yoga for Health Practice Set I are the eye exercises, deep relaxation and Naddi Suddhi.

> *Reality is the leading cause of stress amongst those in touch with it.*
>
> —JANE WAGNER AND LILY TOMLIN

Migraine headaches, precipitated by changes in vascular tension in the blood vessels of the brain, are often brought on by hormone fluctuations during the menstrual cycle. A vegetarian diet may help bring relief for both types of headaches because ease of digestion allows your body's circulation to attend to optimum repair of tension in the nerves, and your hormones will adjust to promote optimal health.

Recommended Asanas

NETHRA VYAYAMAM (EYE EXERCISES)

Relieve eye strain.

MATSYASANA (FISH POSE)

Increases circulation into the cranial nerves situated at the base of the skull, relieving stress and pressure from the vascular system in the brain.

YOGA NIDRA (DEEP RELAXATION)

Allows the spine to relax completely, promoting natural alignment of the vertebrae. Patients with lower-back pain can elevate their legs on a pillow to alleviate stress in the mid-/lower-back muscles. See page 109.

NADDI SUDDHI (ALTERNATE NOSTRIL BREATHING)

Helps to release tension and restore balance to the nervous system.

Allergies
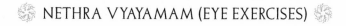

Allergies occur when the body's immune system overreacts to an external substance or to internal imbalance. Why do some people sneeze at pollen, dust, mold and cats while others remain symptom-free? The answer may be related to stress. Foreign substances, called antigens, trigger an antibody reaction that leads to symptoms. Antibodies are proteins produced in the blood to fight off invaders. In an allergic reaction, they end up attacking your own tissues. You can stop this assault by regular practice of the Yoga for Health Practice Set I or II. When your body is deeply relaxed, it can repair defects in the immune system.

> *What we play is life.*
> —LOUIS ARMSTRONG, MUSICIAN

Recommended Asanas

SARVANGASANA (SHOULDERSTAND)

By relaxing the entire system, the Shoulderstand helps to strengthen the immune function, helping to interfere with the antibodies' deleterious assault on the tissues.

KAPALA BATHI (SKULL SHINING)

Increases circulation in the nervous system as well as the lungs, helping to promote relaxation and strengthen the immune system.

MEDITATION

The deep relaxation effect of calming the nervous system is one of the strongest defenses against disease.

Asthma

Asthma occurs when the muscles surrounding the tubes of air going into the lungs become constricted. Emotional stress may affect the degree of tension of these muscles, which are controlled automatically by the brain. Once the muscles become tight, asthmatics have difficulty breathing, and a wheezing sound can be heard. Yoga practice has been documented to relieve and even completely eliminate asthma. The Yoga for Health Practice Sets I and II rebalance the sympathetic (alertness, fight-or-flight) and parasympathetic (relaxation) aspects of the nervous system, relieving stress. Optimum continuing cortisol levels also help explain the success of yoga in treating this condition.

> *Just have faith. If you really give yourself completely in the hands of God, or a Higher Power, you don't have to worry about anything.*
>
> —H.H. Sri Swami Satchidananda

Recommended Asanas

BHUJANGASANA (COBRA POSE)

Opens up the chest, increasing circulation into the lungs. Stimulates the thymus gland and helps in the circulation of white blood cells to the affected area.

DHANYURASANA (BOW POSE)

Opens up the chest, increasing circulation and lymph in that area. Strengthens the membrane lining of the lungs.

JANUSIRASANA (HEAD-TO-KNEE POSE)

Tones the parasympathetic nervous system, helping in the relaxation response.

SARVANGASANA (SHOULDERSTAND)

Brings a fresh blood supply into the lungs and heart.

MATSYASANA (FISH POSE)

Opens the chest, increasing energy, blood and lymph in the lungs and heart.

KAPALA BATHI (SKULL SHINING)

Increases the overall energy of the nerves, glands and organs, helping to strengthen the immune function. Strengthens the lungs.

NADDI SUDDHI (ALTERNATE NOSTRIL BREATHING)

Strengthens, balances and calms the nervous system. Helps to restore lung tissue. *See also* Respiratory System, pages 193–195.

Attention Deficit Disorder (ADD)

ADD, once considered to be a childhood-related condition, affects 4 to 5 percent of American adults, according to a recent article in *USA Today*. Only 15 to 25 percent of those adults know they have it.

Your mind floods with thoughts, causing the inside of your head to sound and feel like the floor of the New York Stock Exchange before the closing bell. You change the subject rapidly and randomly during the course of an ordinary conversation, leaving you and the person you're talking with feeling exhausted, dazed and confused. Other common symptoms of ADD are disorganization, the inability to stay focused or complete projects, frequently losing things, difficulty grasping subject matter and paying attention while reading, memory impairment and lack of impulse control. What are the causes? One prevalent contributing factor is that we are a distractible, multiple task–oriented culture prone to doing several things at the same time. This kind of fragmented mental activity can lead to distracted concentration. Another common demographic at risk for this condition is the remote-control channel surfer. The mental thought processes of a person with ADD are similar to frequent channel flipping. Only, in this case, the frequent flipping is going on in your mind.

According to the Mayo Clinic, a poor diet and a stressful lifestyle can contribute to the onset of ADD by adversely affecting the nervous system and brain chemistry. Because yoga rebalances the glands and organs that affect brain function and the nervous system, it is considered by experts to be a primary adjunctive modality of treatment for ADD. As I have said elsewhere in this book, if you have been diagnosed with a specific medical condition, the poses should be done under the clinical supervision of a physician or other medical professional.

> *Fifty-five percent of all Americans lose their remote control five times a week. That means that they must see the same show for up to three to four minutes at a time!*
>
> —JAY LENO

> *I believe in prayer, I believe in medicine also. Medicine is also a gift from God. Prayer, Hatha yoga practices, medicine and certain dietetic disciplines all could be used at the same time. Even food could be considered a medicine for the pain of hunger. If you believe in prayer, the hunger should just go away. If you eat, then why can't you take medicine also? Prayer and yoga are one form of healing. We can use all the possible ways.*
>
> —H.H. SRI SWAMI SATCHIDANANDA

Recommended Asanas

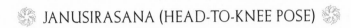 JANUSIRASANA (HEAD-TO-KNEE POSE)

Massages the parasympathetic nervous system (in the lower spine), producing a relaxation effect helpful in the management of anxiety and stress.

SARVANGASANA (SHOULDERSTAND)

The Shoulderstand, done supported or unsupported, is particularly strategic to the sympathetic and parasympathetic nervous systems. Because nerves from the brain go to every tissue of the body, the entire body is dependent on the health of the brain and spine. By increasing blood flow to the scalp and brain, this pose has been clinically observed to promote vitality and increase memory and IQ.

> USA Today *has come out with a new survey—apparently three out of every four people make up 75 percent of the population.*
>
> —David Letterman

MATSYASANA (FISH POSE)

Extends the muscles of the neck and shoulders, helping to increase the space between the vertebrae, allowing them to breathe and alleviating stress in these areas. It also increases circulation to the brain stem and cranial nerves. It should always follow the Shoulderstand.

YOGA NIDRA (DEEP RELAXATION)

By progressively releasing tension from each part of the body and increasing circulation by contracting and releasing the muscles, yoga nidra helps restore the natural health of the body's entire nervous system. When you're lying in the supine position, all the nerves and vertebrae that support the spine and nourish the brain are allowed to "let go" and completely relax, helping to promote spinal alignment and mental balance.

> *I drive too fast to worry about cholesterol.*
>
> —AUTHOR UNKNOWN

KAPALA BATHI (SKULL SHINING)

Because of the "vitality" and "energy" produced by the vigorous repetition of breaths, the entire nervous system is both revitalized and strengthened.

NADDI SUDDHI (ALTERNATE NOSTRIL BREATHING)

By relaxing, purifying and strengthening the subtle nerve currents along the spine and in the brain, alternate nostril breathing has been found to prevent memory loss and restore memory as well as reduce mental and emotional stress.

CARDIOVASCULAR SYSTEM

*C*ardiovascular disease" is a general term for specific conditions related to the heart and circulatory system. It is the number-one cause of death in the United States and in most of the Western world. It is the cause of more deaths than all other diseases combined. For postmenopausal women, heart disease rates are actually higher than for men of the same age due to hormonal and stress factors. This section isolates and describes both common and not-so-common conditions that relate to the cardiovascular system. In order to provide you with a practical understanding of the medical benefits of yoga in the treatment of heart disease, it also includes clinical studies documented by a diverse group of physicians and therapeutic specialists and their patients. Their factual testimonies provide tangible dramatic evidence of how yoga is being used throughout the United States and the world today to fight heart disease.

Richard Gordon, M.A., patient program director for Cedars-Sinai Medical Center Preventive and Rehabilitative Cardiac Center (PRCC), states that the Integral Yoga–based Hatha Yoga Cardiac Program is a vital part of the stress-management

> **PRIMARY ORGAN:** *Heart*
>
> *Related disease conditions*
> Coronary artery disease
> High blood pressure
> Hypertension/Stress
> Cardiomyopathy
> Atrial fibrillation
> Varicose veins
> Angina
> Atherosclerosis
> Congestive heart failure
> Shock

arm of the PRCC. Research over the last several years documents improvements not only in stress reduction but in quality of life for CAD (coronary artery disease) patients. As mentioned previously, the research conducted by Dr. Ornish and Dr. McLanahan has documented that the Integral Yoga–based Yoga for Health program can prevent and reverse heart disease. Published in 1983 in the widely read *Journal of the American Medical Association,* their study, "Effects of Stress Management Training and Dietary Changes in Treating Ischemic Heart Disease," first drew attention to the ability of yoga practice to prevent and reverse cholesterol- and clot-related blockages in the heart's coronary arteries. Their follow-up study "Can Lifestyle Changes Reverse Coronary Heart Disease?" published in the esteemed medical journal *The Lancet,* showed that patients who followed the total yoga program for more than a year exhibited significant improvement in their heart function and vessel constriction, while the coronary blockages of the control group worsened on average.

Continuing studies of patients following the yoga approach have demonstrated a further reduction of coronary plaque in tests performed four to ten years later. Dr.

S. C. Manchanda and associates duplicated this intervention in India, publishing their results, "Retardation of Coronary Atherosclerosis with Yoga Lifestyle Intervention," in the *Journal Association of India* in July 2000. This article described how in a randomized, controlled trial, yoga practice decreased episodes of angina (chest pain), increased exercise capacity, decreased weight, decreased cholesterol and triglyceride levels and helped patients avoid angioplasty and bypass surgery. The research documented an average 20 percent regression of coronary blockage within one year, and reported excellent compliance and no side effects.

Recommended Asanas

JANUSIRASANA (HEAD-TO-KNEE POSE)

CLINICAL NOTE: Postoperative patients should avoid doing this pose if it aggravates the chest area.

Sit on the floor with your legs outstretched. Bring your left heel into the groin area with the sole of your left foot resting against your right inner thigh. Lock your thumbs and raise your arms overhead, stretching your spine up.

Look up at your hands, keep your head aligned between your arms and bend forward over your extended leg. Bring your face to your knee, keeping your leg straight. Relax into the pose. Avoid straining.

Repeat the pose bending over your left leg. Perform once with each leg. Hold for a maximum of ten seconds. See page 99.

Clinical Benefits
Stimulates the parasympathetic nervous system and balances it with the sympathetic nervous system, or the active aspect of that system. It helps to increase blood flow into the coronary arteries.

SARVANGASANA (SHOULDERSTAND): STANDARD VERSION

Adjust your clothing to loosen any restrictions in movement. Lie on your back with your feet together and your arms alongside your body, palms down. Inhale, straighten your legs and lift them over your head in a horizontal position. (If necessary, bend your knees in order to raise them over your head.) Then straighten your legs into a vertical position, keeping them together. Bring your palms to your lower back for support. Begin breathing normally. Keep your chin tucked into your chest. Hold for three minutes. See page 103.

To come out of the pose, lower your legs over your head, parallel to the floor. Bring the arms to the floor for support. Slowly roll the spine to the floor, keeping the legs straight if you can. Otherwise, bend the knees as you come down. Continue breathing normally.

The mental focus in this pose is the base of the throat. Do not sneeze or cough or yawn while in the pose.

SARVANGASANA (SHOULDERSTAND): MODIFIED VERSION

 (a) Lie on your back and elevate your legs to a 90-degree angle. Hold for one to three minutes according to your capacity.
 (b) Lie on your back with your legs elevated on a chair. Hold this position for two to three minutes; come out of the pose sooner if you become uncomfortable.
 (c) Lie on your back with your legs elevated on a wall.

Use these modifications if you have severe high blood pressure, back pain, neck or shoulder injuries or other physiological limitations.

Clinical Benefits

Increases blood flow into the coronary arteries. It stimulates the parasympathetic nervous system and balances it with the sympathetic nervous system, or the active aspect of that system, helping in the treatment of cardiovascular disease, such as cardiomyopathy, CAD (coronary artery disease) and atrial fibrillation. It helps to stablize blood pressure.

YOGA NIDRA (DEEP RELAXATION)

Lie on your back in a comfortable supine position with your arms and legs extended. Your legs should be about a foot and a half apart, and your arms a few inches away from the body with your palms up. Close your eyes and, breathing through your nose, begin relaxing into your position.

Bring your awareness to your right leg and foot. Tense the leg. Lift it off the floor a few inches. Tense a little tighter and let it drop. Roll it from side to side and just forget about it. Repeat with the left leg.

Now inhale and tense your pelvis and buttocks. Squeeze the tension out. Most of us hold a lot of stress in this area, which can lead to disorders in the reproductive system as well as in the pelvis and hips. Now inhale and fill your stomach with air. Hold it for a few moments, then release through your mouth. Just let it gush out.

> *I am still determined to be cheerful and happy, in whatever situation I may be, for I have also learned from experience that the greater part of our happiness or misery depends upon our dispositions, and not upon our circumstances.*
>
> —MARTHA WASHINGTON

Because much of its emphasis is on reducing stress, deep relaxation is considered by physicians such as Dr. McLanahan and Dr. Ornish to be strategic in strengthening and supporting the cardiovascular system.

The guided relaxation has been demonstrated to affect both biochemical and nervous discharge in the direction of a more relaxed state. Blood pressure falls and breathing slows. The process is physiologically more restful than a good night's sleep, yet takes only a few minutes.

DEERGA SWASAM (DEEP BREATHING)

Sit in a cross-legged position, using a wall for support if necessary. Your spine should be erect. Your chest should be expanded, with your shoulders and neck relaxed. Exhale completely. Inhale, filling your abdomen, then your rib cage, then bring the air into your chest. Slowly exhale from your chest, rib cage and abdomen.

Clinical Benefits

Besides maximizing oxygen intake into the blood and all the nerves, organs and glands, this deep breathing practice balances the parasympathetic nervous system located in the lower back, supporting the function of the cardiovascular system.

NADDI SUDDHI (ALTERNATE NOSTRIL BREATHING)

Sit in a comfortable cross-legged position. Make a loose fist with your right hand. Release your thumb and last two fingers. Relax your right arm against your chest and close your right nostril with your right thumb. Slowly exhale as much air as possible without strain through your left nostril. Then inhale through your left nostril and close it with the last two fingers of your right hand. Exhale through your right nostril.

Upon inhalation, be sure to expand your stomach to full capacity to allow as much air as possible to enter your lungs. Upon exhalation, completely empty your lungs. Alternate your breathing this way a few times for as long as is comfortable. Then, have a final exhalation through your right nostril and let your breath return to normal.

Clinical Benefits

Reduces stress from the sympathetic nervous system and balances it with the parasympathetic nervous system, allowing the heart to rest deeply.

Case Study: Cardiomyopathy

Gary Bart, a film producer, is a private heart patient of Dr. Neil Buchbinder, a leading Cedars-Sinai Medical Center cardiologist. He was referred to my Hatha yoga cardiac class at Cedars-Sinai Medical Preventive and Rehabilitative Cardiac Center (PRCC) by Richard Gordon, M.A., the center's patient care manager.

Mr. Bart was admitted to my class in November 2001, with the diagnosis of "idiopathic" cardiomyopathy (weakening of the heart muscle), a form of cardiomyopathy of unknown origin. He presented demonstrating both the subjective and the clinical symptoms of weakness and fatigue. I recommended that he attend the class twice a week. He was given the Integral Yoga–guided relaxation audiotape by Swami Satchidananda and advised to use it a minimum of once a day, between his Hatha yoga cardiac sessions.

In the beginning I monitored Mr. Bart very closely because of the serious and acute nature of his diagnosis and his weakened condition. I restricted his activity in class to the less active modified asanas, omitting the Sun Salutation and requiring him to do the supported Sarvangasana (Shoulderstand) with his legs elevated on a wall. I also cautioned him to come out of a pose, or refrain from doing it altogether, if he felt any degree of strain or uncomfortable symptoms such as undue fatigue, shortness of breath, dizziness, perspiration or nausea.

In spite of his initial misgivings, resistance and skepticism, Mr. Bart proved to be a very disciplined model patient, attending the Hatha yoga cardiac class twice a week with regularity and doing the yoga relaxation as recommended. As a result of his compliance, I began to note a gradual but marked improvement in his condition. Within a month he was exhibiting increased strength, stamina and flexibility, and in between classes he began doing the Hatha yoga cardiac poses on his own, using an instructional videotape. At the end of two months he was allowed to begin participating in the Sun Salutation along with the more advanced members of the class.

During this time he reported personal observations to me, saying he was beginning to experience increased energy and stamina in his daily life, enabling him to begin resuming a more normal lifestyle. While he was also participating in the other critical dynamic modalities in the cardiac program, he specifically remarked that he found the yoga practices to be particularily beneficial and strategic in his progressive recovery process. Besides which, he reported that he really enjoyed doing them.

He continues to attend the class on a regular basis and is fully active and functional in his life and profession.

Physician Testimony

✴ DR. DONNA POLK, M.D. (ASSISTANT DIRECTOR, PRCC)

"Gary Bart began in cardiac rehab when he first noticed symptoms of heart failure as a result of his idiopathic cardiomyopathy. He was having difficulty performing his usual activities because of shortness of breath. Over the last year, Mr. Bart has participated in the integrated cardiac rehabilitation program at PRCC, which includes exercise conditioning, nutrition counseling, group support and yoga. He has increased his exercise tolerance, improved his blood pressure and resting heart rate and can now function normally without symptoms. His participation in the program and particularly his participation in the yoga program have clearly contributed to his functional improvement through the lowering of his blood pressure, improved resting heart rate and improvement in his overall quality of life. Yoga may provide benefit through enhanced parasympathetic tone, thus reducing the risk of adverse events such as sudden cardiac death."

✴ RICHARD GORDON, M.A. (PRCC)

"Yoga is no longer merely an outlier concept for health promotion, but now should be seen as an integral part of any individual's lifestyle for the improvement in their overall health and wellness."

Patient Testimony

✴ GARY BART, FIFTY-FIVE

"I first discovered that I had a problem one Sunday evening in late December 2000. I was sitting, talking to my family, when my heart began to beat wildly. Had I had any coffee? No. Was I excited? No. I didn't give it any more thought and I hoped it would soon disappear. About an hour later it still was going on and I couldn't understand why, so I called my physician. Got the machine and waited for a callback, which never came. About another hour later it was still going on, so I called the hospital. They told me to hang up and call 911, which I did, even though I was not in any pain, nor out of breath or suffering anything except a wildly beating heart. The paramedics took a preliminary cardiogram and rushed me to the hospital. At the ER they tried to diagnose what was going on. Chest X rays, cardiograms, etc. They reviewed the options for getting the heart back to normal rhythm and they chose medications first. After eighteen hours of erratic beating, it finally came back to normal.

"I was told to see the cardiologist for more thorough examinations, stress tests, echo cardiograms, etc., which revealed I had cardiomyopathy. How did I get it? My cardiologist had asked whether I had high blood pressure. Well, I had been treated for high blood pressure for about ten years, but long before that I was very overweight and each doctor's visit showed that my blood pressure was elevated, but he said that all I needed to do was lose weight and it would go down. I didn't lose weight for many years, and so it went untreated. Ten years ago I managed to lose a lot of weight, but still had high blood pressure, so I began taking medication twice a day to reduce it. But, with my busy lifestyle, all too often I forgot to take the medication in the evenings. I had never exercised, so I began working out in the gym, weight training and even hiking on the weekends.

"You know, it's very odd to me that I developed this disease, since obesity runs in my family. My father died of complications of diabetes at the age of fifty-two, and his father from the same thing at age forty-five, so I thought for sure it would be weight-related issues that would get me, not cardiomyopathy. The diagnosis scared me. I tried to find out more about the disease on the Internet, then was sorry I did as it was quite depressing. With my father dying at such a young age, I believed I was doomed.

Humor is tragedy plus time.

—CAROL BURNETT

"My EF (ejection fracture) is around forty now and has been stable for a year, so we're optimistic that we can stabilize it for good. But it took a lot of changing my lifestyle to do that. I started meditating again. I had done TM (transcendental meditation) for about six years in the seventies but hadn't done it since. I entered the Cedars-Sinai Cardiac Rehab program, and joined their Integral Yoga cardiac yoga program that includes Hatha yoga (physical postures), relaxation, meditation and breathing techniques. Me, a former fatty who once weighed 360 pounds, doing yoga? I love it. It gives me such a deep sense of relaxation that seems to build the more I do it.

"When I first began the sessions, I was apprehensive that I would not be able to do any 'wild' poses and wouldn't have the motivation to stay committed to the program. The Integral Yoga method turned out to be a gentle but deeply affecting yoga that I liked instantly. I wasn't aware of the changes at first, as they were subtle. However, I found that I was less frantic, more relaxed and able to handle stress without feeling stressed. I also found that the benefits were increasing as I continued the practice. I began to feel more centered, more able to handle situations that used to baffle me or cause a great deal of stress. No longer was I intimidated by them. And as that happened, I grew in strength, to be able to try new things, and knew that I would be able to handle whatever stress came my way. It's a very fulfilling feeling."

Case Study: Angina Pectoris with Secondary Musculoskeletal and Secondary Abdominal Complaints

Physician Testimony

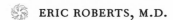 **ERIC ROBERTS, M.D.**

"Mrs. Rottenberg has been attending a Hatha yoga cardiac class given by Nirmala Heriza for about four years. She has benefited from this class; she has lowered her stress and is more relaxed."

Patient Testimony

 ANNA ROTTENBERG

"I have angina pectoris, stomach and back problems. My heart condition was discovered eighteen years ago following an angiogram. At times I was in unbearable pain. Taking medications only helped me to exist.

"Six years ago I began to practice yoga at the suggestion of my occupational therapist. After two months I started feeling much better and my mental state changed. I am having fewer anxiety attacks and my behavior has changed completely. I can take stress without it affecting me. I am sure the yoga nidra deep relaxation plays a big part in these results.

"At first my personal physician was skeptical about my doing yoga for my health, but he has begun to notice a difference in my condition. Although I still take medication, I never miss my yoga practice. Even when I'm out of town."

Case Study: Stress Management

Physician Testimony

DR. JAY NEUFELD, CHAIRMAN OF THE DIVISION OF PEDIATRIC REHABILITATION AT THE MEDICAL COLLEGE OF VIRGINIA, AND DIRECTOR OF PEDIATRIC REHABILITATION AT CHILDREN'S HOSPITAL, RICHMOND, VIRGINIA

"During medical school my yoga practice allowed me to be able to concentrate, to keep my mood more stable, and I didn't feel as fatigued; I emerged energized after each yoga session. I introduced yoga to the American Medical Association, became a vegetarian and became interested in the applications of yoga, diet and nutrition in the treatment and prevention of disease. My experience of the Yoga for Health program in this book further influenced my decision to choose rehabilitation medicine in order to focus on the mind-body connection and a holistic approach to health and illness.

"I happened to be living in New York City during 9/11 and volunteered to serve as a liaison between the New York Medical Center and the morgue. I also helped set up a family crises center and helped in other capacities. Running between the morgue, the families and the hospital, I found the stress beyond words. Yoga classes became the way I kept myself going. I found they were crucially important and allowed me to withstand the almost impossible nature of my work of helping others endure and eventually recover."

Patient Testimony

 MICHEL MOISANT, TWENTY-ONE

"My first exposure to yoga came at the age of seven when, for Christmas, I received a book on yoga for young children. At the time it was a novelty for me. But without any sort of formal guidance, I lost interest and eventually the book receded onto the bookshelf with other childhood literature.

"Years later, in high school, I came across the book again and it piqued my interest in Eastern culture and practices. Again, it started out as a novelty; as a sixteen-year-old I was striving for a more bohemian lifestyle. I began practicing on a regular basis, and while not fully comprehending the benefits at the time, it was something I found I enjoyed doing and provided me with a sense of grounding and stress management I had not found anywhere else.

"Now, as an actor and a student in graduate school, I find myself striving for that same sense of grounding and stress management in every aspect of my life. I have learned the importance of being able to focus energy and channel it in a healthy and productive manner as well as caring for the state of one's body.

"Life is hectic and sometimes my yoga practice falls on my list of priorities. However, the skills of focus and concentration that yoga has taught me are something that I am able to access whether onstage or just trying to get through an unusually busy and stressful day."

Patient Testimony

 MARSHA WENIG

"Back in the seventies and eighties I was a stressed-out professional woman with a succession of careers that included TV news producer, public relations VP, film music coordinator and road manager for the singing group The Manhattan Transfer. My crazy lifestyle led me to yoga, and it proved to be the perfect antidote. Yoga transformed me.

"After having my children I knew I wanted to give them yoga tools at a young age, so maybe they would navigate life's stressors with more ease. My 'playing yoga' with my son and daughter as toddlers, and then in their preschools and eventually their elementary schools, led to the birth of the *YogaKids* program. I'm always tickled and delighted when I leave a school and the children say, 'I wish every day was a yoga day.' *YogaKids* is a stepping-stone on their life's journey. It brings their marvelous inner life to the surface. I watch them shine and feel their brilliance.

"I'm so thankful for yoga and feel gifted to have it be my life's path. *Namaste.*"

Case Study: Hypertension

By clinical definition, hypertension means "high blood pressure," or your systolic blood pressure reading is consistently above 140 and your diastolic is above 90. Prehypertension is when your systolic is between 120 and 130 and your diastolic is consistently between 80 and 89.

According to studies reported by the National Institutes of Health, in the prehypertension stage some kind of lifestyle change or clinical intervention is recommended to bring blood pressure back to normal—120/80 or below.

High blood pressure is commonly recognized as a precursor to heart attack and strokes. Both diet and stress are key factors in heart attacks and strokes, however there can be secondary causes rooted in other systemic disorders such as kidney disease or conditions related to the adrenal glands.

When you make the finding yourself— even if you're the last person on Earth to see the light—you'll never forget it.

—CARL SAGAN, PHYSICIST

Since up to 80 percent of illness is stress-related, yoga's ability to help patients reduce the effects of stress in their lives is central to healing.

Dr. Herbert Benson, a researcher at Harvard University, conducted studies to show that regular meditation alone can be utilized as an effective treatment for hypertension. In 1972 he published the results of his work in the prestigious medical journal *Circulation* in an article entitled "Decreased Blood Pressure in Hypertensive Subjects Who Practiced Meditation."

In 1969, Dr. K. K. Datey showed the effectiveness of yoga nidra (deep relaxation)—an element of the Yoga for Health program—in lowering blood pressure.

He announced his results in the publication *Antiology* in an article entitled "Reductions in Blood Pressure Using Yoga Deep Relaxation." The Yoga for Health restorative yoga program is based on *all* aspects of yoga and is therefore even more effective in treating hypertension and stress-related disorders than its discrete elements.

Physician Testimony

DR. MEHMET OZ, CARDIOLOGIST, DIRECTOR OF THE COLUMBIA PRESBYTERIAN MEDICAL CENTER'S HEART-ASSIST DEVICE PROGRAM AND COFOUNDER AND MEDICAL DIRECTOR OF ITS PIONEERING COMPLEMENTARY CARE CENTER. DR. OZ IS AUTHOR OF *HEALING FROM THE HEART*.

"I use yoga as means of dealing with my own physical strain as well as the stress of my patients. Because of doing yoga, I am not plagued by the orthopedic issues most surgeons face from being cramped over an operating table all day. In addition, whenever I feel stressed in any aspect of my life, I turn to yoga to help relieve my tension; it's the best way I know to calm my mind. It acts to condition awareness, keeping you loose and ready for the inevitable challenges of the day."

Dr. Oz suggests that every one of his patients do yoga before surgery, and afterward. As he says, "It helps to prevent the lung problems and lack of flexibility that can occur after an operation, especially common when we are operating on the main axis of the body. The asanas included in Yoga for Health help diminish pain, ensure a quicker recovery and act preventively, postoperatively. Yoga has been one of the most commonly used modalities for patients and physicians in the Columbia-Presbyterian Heart Institute."

Physician Testimony

DR. SANDRA MCLANAHAN

"D.D. is a forty-four-year-old African-American businessman and restaurateur who comes from a family with a history of chronic high blood pressure. The stresses of his various enterprises, the ups and downs of the economy and a difficult divorce had begun to contribute to headaches, chronic fatigue and his feeling generally out of shape.

"On examination, his blood pressure was 185/125. Instead of going on medication, he chose to first follow the total health yoga program. He began doing daily yoga practice, which he noticed immediately began to relieve his symptoms of headaches and fatigue. He focused on doing all of the postures, but particularly felt benefit from the Sun Salutation, the Cobra and the Head-to-Knee poses. His blood pressure was lowered within two weeks to 125/84.

"He also changed to a vegetarian-based diet, eliminating meat, cheese and sweet drinks. He began drinking only water, eating breakfast regularly and replacing white flour and white sugar with moderate amounts of complex carbohydrates, such as oatmeal and brown rice. His weight gradually dropped from 250 pounds to 212 pounds over a six-month period.

"D.D. now maintains his new healthy lifestyle, averaging blood pressures less than 120/80, and has experienced a renewed exuberance that has been noticed by friends and family. He feels that he is addressing his familial risk factors and is now intent on educating the African-American community, which is at special risk for hypertension and heart disease because of stress and a high-fat diet."

Case Study: Hypertension/Myocardial Infarction (Heart Attack)

Physician Testimony

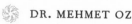 **DR. MEHMET OZ**

"A fifty-five-year-old patient of mine who worked as a football coach was keeping his team overtime, pushing them and himself to the limit. Often, to his friends and family, he would say, 'This game is going to kill me.' Then one day he suddenly felt crushing chest pain, became cold and sweaty and felt pain radiating down his left arm. He thought he must finally be having a heart attack and asked to be taken to the hospital. But he also thought to himself, 'Just in case it isn't, let me grab my cigarettes.'

"When I confirmed that, indeed, it was a heart attack and he would need bypass surgery, I recommended that he do yoga practices to prepare for and recover from the operation. 'I'm not into that BS, just operate,' was my patient's response.

"I decided to use yoga as an analogy for preparing for a football game. I asked him, 'Don't you get mentally prepared, do some exercises and get your game face on? This is the way to thrive in the game of heart surgery, to get mentally ready. And these are the pre-practice exercises.'

"By using this metaphor, the patient understood. I helped him gain insight into the advantages of using this form of preparation, and thus he began doing yoga. The coach discovered that some of the asanas were similar to the stretches he was using to limber up his football players. He found that many sports teams, such as the Los Angeles Lakers, now incorporate yoga into their warm-up routines. As an added benefit, the coach found that the yoga practices helped him to finally quit smoking. He now continues to do a regular yoga routine to help prevent heart problems in the future."

Case Study: Atrial Fibrillation

Clinician Testimony

❋ **NIRMALA HERIZA, BA, CYT**

"S.M.T. has been a patient of mine since 1992. She was referred to me by my physician colleague Dr. Ornish, who recommended I begin treating her atrial fibrillation with the restorative yoga program for cardiac patients. He also suggested I refer her to the director of cardiac rehabilitation at Cedars-Sinai Medical Center, Dr. Noel Bairey Merz, for additional medical supervision. Dr. Merz corroborated Dr. Ornish's recommendation for cardiac yoga.

"At first the patient reported that she was very depressed and fatigued. She was very weakened by her condition and concerned that she would never go a day without an episode of atrial fibrillation. In particular, she was afraid that one day her heart would be in permanent fibrillation.

"While I saw her twice a week for the regular restorative Yoga for Health program, I suggested she do just the yoga nidra (relaxation) and pranayama on her own every day. Gradually, she built up her stamina to where she was doing the yoga postures at least twice a week on her own in addition to her supervised sessions. She also began increasing her regular walking exercise activity. Clinically, she began to demonstrate stabilizing factors.

"In general, in addition to her positive response, she is now clinically more stable, stronger and much more vital than when she first began cardiac yoga therapy with me. Even though, due to various stressful variables, S.M.T. has experienced periodic episodes of atrial fibrillation, the yoga practices have brought her out of the trauma and helped to stabilize her condition on a more regular basis. Daily Naddi Suddhi breathing, in particular, has been instrumental in stabilizing these AF episodes. Both Dr. Ornish and Dr. Merz are very pleased with my progress reports on how her condition has been ameliorated."

Patient Testimony

S.M.T.

"When I was thirty-seven years old I was diagnosed with mitral valve prolapse. Since the early 1990s I have had episodes of atrial fibrillation. I wasn't walking on a regular basis and was not on any kind of meditation program to treat my condition. I consulted with Dr. Dean Ornish, who recommended yoga as an adjunct therapy for my symptomatology of stress and fatigue and referred me to his Los Angeles associate, Nirmala Heriza, to supervise my practice. My sister had also been a participant in Dr. Ornish's Program for Reversing Heart Disease and was very enthusiastic about doing yoga as a means of relaxation.

"I take life very seriously and am under a great deal of stress. Since beginning the Integral Yoga–based cardiac therapy with Ms. Heriza, my life has changed tremendously. I have become more limber, my vitality has increased and my episodes of atrial fibrillation are not as frequent and don't last as long. On one recent weekend I had an episode that was more prolonged than usual. I was preparing to see my cardiologist on Monday to have my heart 'controverted' back into normal sinus rhythm. He scheduled me for the clinic on Wednesday. In the meantime, after conferring with Dr. Ornish, Ms. Heriza recommended that in the interim I do yoga postures and in particular the Naddi Suddhi (alternate nostril breathing) three times a day. I followed their suggestion and on Tuesday my heart 'controverted' itself into sinus rhythm without the help of intervention. This was the first time this had ever happened on its own, without clinical cardioversion. My doctor had me undergo an EKG, which confirmed that my heart was beating regularly, and he sent me home.

"I am hyperkalemic (too much postassium) and my cholesterol and homocysteine levels are low, so my diet is very restricted. I have found that eating a low-fat diet and exercising are important in managing my health, but the yoga and pranayama techniques are vital. If it weren't for these natural remedies, I believe I would be in permanent atrial fibrillation.

"Physicians I've consulted with subsequently have told me that it is amazing that my heart has remained in sinus rhythm for so long. I owe it to Ms. Heriza and Dr. Ornish for recommending that I adhere strictly to a regular practice of yoga, and do Naddi Suddhi at least three times a day to keep my heart rate stable.

I have found relaxation and meditation to be the most important elements of the Yoga for Health program. I know this type of yoga and this program have saved my life."

Spinal-Skeletal/ Musculo-Ligamentous System

The musculoskeletal system provides form, stability and movement to the human body. It consists of the body's bones (which make up the skeleton), muscles, tendons, ligaments, joints, cartilage and other connective tissue. The "connective tissue" (fascia) is the fibrous tissue that binds other tissues and organs together. Its chief components are elastic fibers and collagen, a protein substance. Connective tissue provides support to the various structures of the body—it holds organs in place and provides the underlying structure for all tissues. The yoga asanas stretch, massage and promote circulation, mobility and vitality in this system and all its many parts. The stretching of the joints in the asanas produces secretion of synovial fluid, a lubricant released into the joints that keeps them supple and removes waste products. The result is to reduce stiffness, which prevents arthritis and other joint-related conditions.

The Mayo Clinic, a venerated medical institution, recently began to endorse yoga as a treatment for various serious medical conditions. As reported in the clinic's September 2003 newsletter, clinical study shows that in the treatment of

AREAS AFFECTED

Cervical spine

Cervical paraspinals: splenius cervicus, splenius

Levator scapula

Trapezius muscles

Thoracic spine

Intercostal muscles

Supraspinatus muscle

Infraspinatus muscle

Scapula

Teres muscle

Teres minor

Upper extremities

Deltoid bursa

Brachioradialis

Carpal

Lumbar spine

Erector spinae muscles

Quadradus luborum

Iliolumbar spine

Piriformis muscle

Gluteus muscles

Related disease conditions

General tightness of the fascia of the neck,
    mid and lower back

Arthritis

Muscular strain

Temporomandibular joint syndrome (TMJ)

> Frozen shoulder syndrome
>
> Bursitis
>
> Kyphosis (rounding of the upper spine)
>
> Lordosis (inversion of the lower spine)
>
> Osteoporosis
>
> Carpal tunnel syndrome
>
> Sciatica
>
> Low back syndrome

carpal tunnel syndrome—a painful condition of the wrist joints—people who use yoga and relaxation techniques in addition to wearing a wrist splint experience more relief than people who use the splint alone. Another study in the same publication revealed that people with osteoarthritis of the hands who took yoga classes had less finger pain and tenderness than those who didn't take yoga classes.

Recommended Asanas

SURYA NAMASKARAM (SUN SALUTATION)

Stretches the entire body, increasing circulation into the heart, lungs and all the major organs, muscles and joints. It tones the major muscle groups and promotes spinal alignment and flexibility, rejuvenating the nervous system. It stimulates the endocrine system, helping to support the immune function. It is beneficial in the prevention and treatment of arthritis by promoting the secretion of synovial fluid in the joints. For cardiac patients, it promotes cardiovascular circulation. See page 93.

✸ ARDDHASALABASANA (HALF LOCUST) ✸

Strengthens the back, pelvis and abdomen, helping in the treatment of lower-back weakness, tightness and spasm. The disk space between the spinal vertebrae is stretched, helping to promote spinal alignment. The sympathetic nervous system (the portion of the nervous system devoted to arousal for fight or flight, located in the mid back) is balanced, helping in the treatment of heart disease. Pressure increases in the heart and lungs, helping their elasticity and lymph drainage. It increases circulation and massages the prostate or uterus and ovaries and is therefore helpful in the treatment of prostate or uterine disease. See page 98.

✸ YOGA NIDRA (DEEP RELAXATION) ✸

Allows the spine to relax completely, promoting natural alignment of the vertebrae. Patients with lower-back pain can elevate their legs on a pillow to alleviate stress in the mid-/lower-back muscles. See page 109.

✸ KAPALA BATHI (SKULL SHINING) ✸

Strengthens the mid-/lower-back muscles and nerves. See page 28.

✸ NADDI SUDDHI (ALTERNATE NOSTRIL BREATHING) ✸

Allows the spine to relax completely, promoting the natural alignment of the vertebrae. Patients with lower-back pain can elevate their legs on a pillow to ease pressure on the paraspinals (the muscles along the spine). See page 111.

Case Study: Back Pain

Chronic back pain is one of the most common health problems Americans have. More than 80 percent of us have significant problems with our backs during our lifetimes. Under physical or mental stress, muscles tighten and produce more lactic acid, a by-product of muscle work. This acid acts as an irritant, and the muscles contract even further. As a result, we feel musculoskeletal pain and discomfort. The conventional, drug-oriented approach to this problem is the use of muscle relaxants or pain relievers, which may leave you feeling sedated or afflicted by serious side effects such as stomach ulcers or addiction.

The Yoga for Health restorative program promotes a gentle, localized increase in circulation, which helps to change your tight muscles and ligaments into a more elastic, relaxed state, which in turn helps free you of pain.

Physician Testimony

 DR. RANDY VAN NOSTRAND, M.D.

"My interest in yoga as a treatment regime began with my own injured back. During a high-stress time of going through a divorce, I was hit by a drunk driver, resulting in debilitating distress in my back. Two failed papain injections left me with a back stiffer than ever as well as constant pain. I began the Yoga for Health program recommended in this book and became completely free of discomfort for the first time in ten years. I then started using the yoga approach with my patients in Tucson, Arizona, and witnessed significant pain relief and reversal of musculoskeletal disease. Next I invented a way to do yoga in my pool while floating in a small inner tube, aided by a neck pillow and ankle weights. I named my approach Aqua-yoga and found it exceptionally helpful for my patients with back disease, especially for those who at first were not comfortable doing the yoga practices on dry land."

Patient Testimony

ANNIE APPLEBY

"A little more than a decade ago, when I was working at Paramount Pictures as a legal liaison in Hollywood, I began taking a yoga class on the studio lot to unwind. I hated my first yoga class. I am a Type A marathon runner. At first, the class seemed slow and boring, but to my surprise I felt great afterward and I was told by Marion Stork, the yoga instructor, to 'give the yoga a chance, three times a week for two weeks. If you do not feel benefits and see results, then you do not need to ever try it again.'

"I started loving it. I saw results fast and never stopped. In fact, yoga changed my life. I lost ten pounds permanently; I ate healthier food and eliminated red meat from my diet. I learned to listen to my body and keep it running efficiently. Yoga affected me in the mindful ways as well. I could feel yoga was a tremendous healer.

"I live in LA and I drive a lot. I have been in my share of bumper-thumpers. The last one was so bad, my orthopedic surgeon told me I would never be able to run again. He said to continue yoga because it was very 'healing.' That was four years ago. Now, thanks to yoga, I can run marathons again. I am also an inch taller.

"I decided that everyone should do yoga, and I wanted to help get the word out. In 1995 I cashed out my savings and created Yoga Force, registered the name and sold the clothing line I had designed, without any training in the field whatsoever, to over 150 stores in the U.S. I have also placed the clothes and accessories in TV shows and films, including one of Arnold Schwarzenegger's *Terminator* films.

"If everyone did yoga, the world would be a much better place. I believe that now more than ever."

Case Study: Plantar Fasciitis (Inflammation of the Tendons of the Feet)

Patient Testimony

✿ **LINDSAY CROUSE**

"When I consulted with Nirmala Heriza for Integral Yoga Hatha and myofascial (soft tissue muscle) therapy, I was in a desperate state of mind. I had severe plantar fasciitis, inflammation of the tendons that run under the feet. The tugging of these tendons over the years had caused two large bone spurs to appear under my heels. On the X ray they looked like pruning hooks. I was hobbled. The pain kept up even when I wasn't walking. I had resorted to cortisone shots and had been told by more than one doctor that the only cure was to sever the tendon, an operation that to me was too frightening to contemplate.

"Nirmala suggested I do the Travell myofascial therapy to break down the fasciitis, or crystallized particles, in the tendons, and acupressure and yoga to increase circulation, stretch the tendons and reduce my stress associated with the condition.

"At first, the whole thing seemed naive. I thought I needed something to replace the drugs and surgery. I needed to bring in the big guns. I had done acupuncture, taken herbs, dabbled in ayurvedic medicine, swallowed potions with ground-up beetles in them. Nothing had touched this injury. But Nirmala said she had successfully treated several patients with my diagnosis who had been referred to her by podiatrists. She seemed confident, medically informed and at ease about it, so I said, 'OK, let's do it.' As a result of the yoga, combined with the other physical therapy techniques she did with me three times a week for three months, my plantar fasciitis has improved to where I can resume my regular activities. Today my feet are flexible and pain-free."

Case Study: Carpal Tunnel Syndrome

Carpal tunnel syndrome is a very common condition that affects millions of Americans today. Many people in professions requiring repetitive use of the hands, such as computer operators, butchers, machinery operators and piano and tennis players, are at a high risk of developing this condition.

The carpal tunnel is situated at the base of the palm. The floor and walls of the tunnel are formed by the carpal bones of the wrist, and the carpal ligament forms the roof. The median nerve and nine flexor tendons pass through the tunnel. The median nerve, which runs from the neck to the fingertips, governs thumb strength and feeling in the thumb, index, middle and part of the ring finger. If overuse or injury causes swelling of the tissues in the carpal tunnel, the median nerve becomes compressed, leading to pain and weakness of the fingers.

In 1999, Dr. W. Seurian published an article in the medical journal *The Lancet* entitled "Yoga in the Treatment of Carpal Tunnel Syndrome." In the article he showed that yoga is an effective therapeutic approach to both treating and preventing this condition. He found that yoga "worked even better than splinting the wrist." Dr. M. S. Garfinkel, whose paper "A Yoga-Based Intervention for Carpal Tunnel Syndrome" appeared in 1998 in the *Journal of the American Medical Association*, likewise showed that a total yoga intervention can reverse this painful problem.

ENDOCRINE SYSTEM

*T*he endocrine system is governed by a group of tactical underground chemical messengers called "hormones," which help to carry out a wide variety of physiological processes. These hormones regulate metabolism, growth and sexual development. The endocrine glands release hormones directly into the bloodstream, where they are transported to the organs and tissues throughout the body. The most vital glands of this system are the pituitary, pineal, thyroid, adrenal, pancreas and sex glands. The pituitary and pineal glands are situated in the brain. The thyroid is in the neck region; the adrenals and pancreas are in the solar plexus (abdominal) area; the sex glands are in the pelvic region. If you respect and care for them, they, in turn, will be your most reliable friends.

The yoga postures act to optimize circulation through the endocrine glands. This allows them to perform more effectively in their maintenance and repair functions, so that any inflammation, under- or overactive functioning or hormone imbalance can be more efficiently addressed by the body's self-regulatory mechanisms.

PRIMARY ORGANS

Pineal gland

Pituitary gland

Thyroid gland

Pancreas

Liver

Spleen

Kidneys

Adrenal glands

Prostate gland

Uterus

Related disease conditions

AIDS

Prostate cancer

Ovarian cancer

Diabetes

Leukemia

Breast cancer

Obesity

Hasimoto's thyroiditis (underactive thyroid)

Graves' disease (overactive thyroid)

Urinary tract disease

Related disease conditions such as infection, AIDS and cancer may also be more appropriately tackled by the immune system when circulatory enhancement and rebalancing of the body's nervous systems of excitement and relaxation (sympathetic and parasympathetic nervous systems) take place.

Recommended Asanas

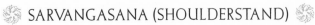 SARVANGASANA (SHOULDERSTAND)

Regulates the thyroid gland and stabilizes the metabolism; helpful in the treatment of overactive and underactive thyroid conditions. Stimulates the baroreceptors in the neck, lowering blood pressure and pulse rate.

> *Health is the greatest gift, contentment, the greatest wealth, faithfulness the best relationship.*
>
> —THE BUDDHA

Balances the sympathetic and parasympathetic nervous systems, further helping to support the cardiovascular system. Stimulates the pineal and pituitary glands in the center of the brain, thereby balancing the sympathetic and parasympathetic nervous systems. Because of the increased blood and lymph drainage toward the upper body, when you stand up again the improved flow of these fluids into your legs and lower organs provides relief for varicose veins and hemorrhoids—conditions that result from the excessive pressure of gravity on the valves in the veins. See pages 102–104.

MATSYASANA (FISH POSE)

Increases circulation to the lungs. As reported by the *Journal of the American Medical Association* (*JAMA*), the Fish Pose has been clinically recognized to be effective in treating a variety of conditions. By extending the cervical and thoracic spine backward, the neck and upper back and chest muscles are stretched and stimulated, increasing flexibility and circulation. Because it improves circulation to the thyroid, this pose helps the gland regulate itself so that it is neither over- nor underactive, thereby stabilizing metabolism. It also increases blood flow to the cardiovascular system, helping in the prevention and treatment of heart disease. See page 104.

✵ YOGA NIDRA (DEEP RELAXATION) ✵

Relieves strain and tightness of the lower back. It massages the abdominal organs and digestive tract, increasing circulation and pushing the contents of the bowel along, helping to relieve constipation. Any accumulated gas can also be expelled, thus relieving the pressure of flatulence. See page 109.

✵ NADDI SUDDHI (ALTERNATE NOSTRIL BREATHING) ✵

Balances the sympathetic (active) and parasympathetic (relaxation response) nerves, thereby strengthening the endocrine glands. See page 111.

Case Study: Obesity

The current obesity epidemic has reached truly alarming proportions. Its pervasiveness has been matched by the glut of diet schemes and exercise regimes feverishly embraced in mostly frustratingly futile attempts to conquer the weight-gain dragon—an effort that seems to drag on and on.

Dr. Ornish and Dr. McLanahan's research with heart disease patients has produced an important side benefit that can help with the struggle to control weight. Their research

> *Never eat more than you can lift.*
> —Miss Piggy

shows that a very low-fat, high-fiber diet combined with daily yoga practices such as those in the Yoga for Health program described in this book not only prevents and reverses heart disease and cancer but helps people reach and maintain their appropriate weight, with an astonishing 70 to 90 percent success rate.

No other weight-loss regime has had anywhere near this success, and none has had the rigorous scientific long-term investigation to substantiate its effectiveness.

The in-depth research describing this program is summarized in Dr. Ornish's book *Eat More, Weigh Less,* which reached number one on *The New York Times* bestseller list.

This yoga-based approach is not just another fad. Instead of merely focusing on weight loss, it emphasizes the lifestyle choices that are best for keeping your body free from illness in the long term. The combination of the Hatha yoga practices and dietary recommendations provides the very best comprehensive system for maintaining and sustaining a healthy lifestyle.

Daily yoga practice is essential to any approach to weight loss because its calming effect assists you in sticking to a diet. Yoga helps reverse the buildup of stress in the muscles and keeps you more relaxed during the day, which makes you less likely to choose inappropriate foods or overeat as you struggle to lose weight.

Physician Testimony

DR. SANDRA MCLANAHAN

"Chronic stress itself can cause excess secretion of the adrenal hormone cortisol, which encourages the body to store fat, especially around the waistline. Daily yoga stretches and relaxation have been documented to result in lower baseline cortisol levels. Yoga practice also increases the body's levels of serotonin, endorphins and dopamine, chemicals associated with feelings of serenity and tranquillity, giving you strength to resist the doughnuts and junk food in the well-stocked supermarkets.

> *Only I can change my life, no one can do it for me.*
>
> —CAROL BURNETT, ACTRESS, COMEDIAN

"Yoga has been shown to balance right-left brain activity toward states of more calm and feelings of more control. Increased activity in the limbic system, the brain's emotional center, is also accompanied by an elevated number of theta brain waves, associated with the relaxed state of pre-sleep. Sleep deprivation itself, by increasing cortisol levels, has been shown to be associated with obesity, and yoga practice can help in overcoming the common problem of insomnia as well.

"Obesity itself is a separate risk factor for high blood pressure, diabetes, heart disease, arthritis and cancer. Thus, it is worth making a concerted effort to reach and continue at a more ideal weight. Acting to control this massive challenge can help avoid many problems down the road. Daily yoga may seem difficult at first, but step by step, as flexibility of both body and mind increases, so does a real solution to the obstacles of achieving and maintaining your optimum weight."

Patient Testimony

 J.R., SIXTY-FIVE

"I not only carried excess weight, but suffered from stiffness, shortness of breath on exertion and sleep apnea. My big 'spare tire' got in my way a lot, but I just couldn't discipline myself enough to stay on a diet. Losing weight alone was just not enough of a motivation. However, after commencing this yoga program, I began to enjoy it so much that I was motivated to lose that waist bulge so I could do the forward-bend yoga postures better.

"I lost thirty pounds, my midsection became normal, and my shortness of breath and sleep apnea disappeared. I felt so much better that I even went mountain climbing, in the course of which I did much more than participants twenty years younger than me. When they found themselves short of breath at the high altitude, I ended up helping them up the slopes."

> *If you have total faith in a Higher Will—a Higher Energy—you will be able to tune in to that and receive all the strength and energy to recharge your system.*
>
> —H.H. SRI SWAMI SATCHIDANANDA

Physician Testimony

DR. SANDRA MCLANAHAN

"In addition to being overweight, R.D., a forty-eight-year-old woman, suffered from disproportionate distribution of the weight: her waist, hips and thighs were excessively bulging. She had difficulty walking and sitting. The first thing she noticed after she began her daily yoga practice was that gradually the weight began to be more appropriately distributed, and her shape and form began to change. She also began walking better, and her posture improved. After one year she had accomplished a twenty-pound weight loss, which she has maintained. She now teaches yoga, is in great shape, her proportions are excellent, and she looks and feels much better."

IMMUNE SYSTEM

He that takes medicine and neglects diet, wastes the skill of the physician.

—CHINESE PROVERB

I stand in awe of my body.

—HENRY DAVID THOREAU

Stay in your true Self. You are the knower. You know everything. When you are happy you know you are happy. When you suffer you know you suffer. This knowing is permanent. You know you have a headache, but at the same time you say, "I am aching." This identification should be avoided. When you mix yourself up with your identifications and possessions, pull yourself out of the mire and your feelings will change greatly. You'll be a different person.

—H.H. SRI SWAMI SATCHIDANANDA, *THE YOGA SUTRAS OF PATANJALI*

As mentioned in Part I the body's immune system is central to its overall health. It's your body's fortress. Its tactical defense mechanisms detect invaders and protect the body and its organs and systems from them, whether they are toxins or disease-causing agents such as bacteria and viruses. When functioning properly, the immune system prevents chronic diseases, fights infections and increases longevity.

There are two primary ways the immune system begins to malfunction. First, by

PRIMARY ORGANS

Bone marrow
Thymus
Spleen
Lymph nodes
Liver

Related disease conditions
Cancer
Allergies
Fibromyalgia
Hepatitis
Arthritis
Juvenile diabetes
Diabetes
Rheumatoid arthritis
Multiple sclerosis
Chronic fatigue
Chron's disease
Anemia
Addison's disease

overreacting to a substance that normally isn't a threat such as pollen, causing an allergic reaction, or to substances that cause arthritis or lupus. Second, it can weaken and fail to react appropriately, thus allowing the growth of cancerous cells, the spread of herpes viruses or the development of conditions such as chronic fatigue syndrome. It also predisposes the system to less serious conditions such as colds and the flu.

The major organs of the immune system are dispersed throughout the body.

They include the lymph nodes (situated in groups along lymphatic vessels), bone marrow (in the core of the bones), the thymus (in the upper part of the chest) and the spleen (on the left side of the abdomen). These organs produce and store an array of white blood cells and specialized immune cells. These cells help the body detect invading agents, produce antibodies that neutralize or destroy them, turn off the immune reaction when it is no longer needed and store the process in their memory for future reference.

> *The Remedy often proves worse than the disease.*
>
> —WILLIAM PENN

K. H. Coker, an eminent medical researcher, relates, "There is evidence of the effect of yoga/meditation on melatonin, a hormone produced by the pineal gland, which may affect breast and prostate tumors. A preliminary study finds an association between yoga/meditation practice and levels of melatonin."

In 2003 Dr. Barry Oken, M.D., neurology professor at Oregon Health and Science University, documented significant improvement in the fatigue levels of sixty-nine patients with MS after they began a yoga program.

The yoga asanas in the Yoga for Health restorative program balance and promote circulation into specific glands and organs so they can more efficiently do their work in helping to treat chronic disease.

Recommended Asanas

 SARVANGASANA (SHOULDERSTAND)

(To be done either supported or unsupported)

Regulates the thyroid gland and stabilizes the metabolism; helpful in the treatment of overactive or underactive thyroid conditions. Stimulates the baroreceptors in the neck, lowering blood pressure and pulse rate. Stimulates the pineal and pituitary glands in the center of the brain, thereby balancing the sympathetic and parasympathetic nervous systems and futher helping in the treatment of immune-related disorders such as cancer, chronic fatigue, AIDS and the flu (see also Common Ailments, page 115). See pages 102–104.

🌸 MATSYASANA (FISH POSE) 🌸

Because it improves circulation to the thyroid, the Fish Pose helps this gland regulate itself so that it is neither over- nor underactive, thereby stabilizing metabolism.

It increases blood flow into the cardiovascular system, helping support various glands and organs such as the thymus gland (in the chest above the heart) and spleen (in the right upper abdomen), helping the white blood cells that make up the immune system circulate and target infection. See page 104.

> *Faith is the strength by which a shattered world shall emerge into the light.*
>
> —HELEN KELLER

🌸 YOGA NIDRA (DEEP RELAXATION) 🌸

By helping you relax deeply, this pose strengthens and reinforces the immune system and helps the body fight infection and disease. See page 109.

NADDI SUDDHI
(ALTERNATE NOSTRIL BREATHING)

Balances the sympathetic and parasympathetic nervous systems. Strengthens the pineal and thymus glands and the spleen. This activity promotes white blood cell activity and helps to reinforce the immune system. See page 111.

Case Study: Cancer

Since 1970, statistics have increasingly demonstrated the possibility that exists for all age demographics to survive cancer and ameliorate the therapeutic residuals. Testimonies by many recovering patients and survivors bear witness to this fact. The verified clinical information presented in this book is strong evidence of how this challenge is being met with stunning results. It is also an unequivocal statement of how far conventional medicine has come in recognizing and implementing yoga and other alternative protocols as legitimate medical adjunct modalities.

> *Misdirected lifeforce is the activity in the disease process.*
>
> —KABBALAH

In an article entitled "Mindfulness-based Stress Reduction in Relation to Quality of Life, Mood, Symptoms of Stress, and Immune Parameters in Breast and Prostate Cancer Patients," published in *Psychosomatic Medicine* in July 2003, Dr. L. Carlson and colleagues documented that meditation practice increases overall quality of life, decreases symptoms of stress and improves sleep quality as well as increases specific immune factors such as IL-4, thought to be associated with the body's ability to destroy cancer cells. The blood changes fit the picture of a relatively depressed immune system returning to normal.

Clinical Testimony

In 1976 Michael Lerner, Ph.D., founded the cancer-help organizations Commonweal, in Bolinas, California, in 1996 and sister organization Smith Farm Center for the Healings Arts, in Washington, D.C., to help cancer patients empower themselves. Patients learn yoga and other gentle therapies and share their experiences in a group setting. Week-long retreats are the regular format.

> *One who gains strength by overcoming obstacles, possesses the only strength which can overcome adversity.*
>
> —ALBERT SCHWEITZER, M.D.

These centers have successfully showed that cancer patients' sense of relaxation, relief from pain and quality of life can be significantly improved by doing the yoga practices. Shanthi Norris, Executive Director of the Smith Farm Center, was quoted in *The Washington Post* in November 2000: "Our humble goal is to help transform the medical community." She teaches the program's yoga classes and has witnessed their ability to help cancer patients cope.

❀ LESLIE BOGART, R.N.

"As a registered nurse I worked with very ill patients in an intensive care unit setting. I treated them as required, talked with them and their families as needed. As a yoga teacher I work therapeutically with students who are beginners who have injuries or diseases. In my experience yoga helps people with normal life stresses as well as those with severe pain or potentially life-threatening conditions. The practice of asanas and pranayama offers balance and support as well as strength and flexibility. Releasing tensions in the body and calming the mind with yoga help people who are undergoing chemotherapy or who have a serious illness go through treatment and live more comfortably. Strengthening, stretching and learning to move without causing more pain to an already inflamed area can help reduce and sometimes eliminate pain.

Life is about not knowing, having to change, taking the moment and making the best of it without knowing what's going to happen next.

—GILDA RADNER

"My personal yoga practice has given me tools for myself as well as for my students to find calm, wisdom and support, thus enhancing and improving their life experience."

Case Study: Uterine Cancer

Physician Testimony

❀ DR. BOUCHAIB RABBANI, PH.D.

"Marion was diagnosed with uterine cancer in 1991 and underwent a surgical procedure to remove the cancer. A peritoneal wash was done to find if the cancer had spread to her peritoneum, and it had. She received chemotherapy treatments to eradicate the free-floating cancerous cells. Her surgical oncologist recently gave her a clean bill of health.

"After her surgery Marion followed a strict regimen of yoga, meditation and healthy living. I'm sure this helped her overcome any remaining cancer cells."

Patient Testimony

 MARION TAYLOR

"On December 18, 2002, I went for my annual gynecological exam. For the first time in eleven years, my doctor finally said that I am cured of cancer. He said, 'As of today, you're coming for well-woman exams and no longer as a cancer patient, for my insurance code purposes.' To hear him say this was like a great blessing.

Lots of people want to ride with you in the limo. But what you want is someone who will take the bus with you when the limo breaks down.

—OPRAH WINFREY

"As I think back, memories flood my mind of incredible fear and stunned disbelief from the day when I was diagnosed with a rare and very aggressive uterine cancer. Then there was the worry after surgery, waiting in my bed at Memorial Hospital in Long Beach for several days for the results of the washings in my body cavity to determine if there were any stray cancer cells . . . and there were. I was placed on a radioactive liquid treatment as an alternative to chemo or radiation, and it proved to be successful for me.

"In follow-up checkups with Dr. Berman, he commented on how quickly I had recovered from my surgery. I attribute it to the restorative yoga poses, prayer and positive affirmations, and vitamin therapy prescribed by Dr. McLanahan.

"My guru, Swami Satchidananda, would always say, 'You are what you think.' During my recovery I listened daily to healing affirmations and relaxation tapes, and meditated regularly. I had to begin doing Hatha yoga again slowly because of the scar tissue. I did the easy, modified restorative poses. I did my best to remain peaceful and would visualize my body being healed. I did not think of myself as a sick person or as a cancer patient.

Don't deny the diagnosis; try to deny the verdict.

—NORMAN COUSINS

"Finally, when I got stronger, I followed my heart and went back to college part-time to study design. Even though I had gone back to work, I think school kept my mind focused on something really positive to look forward to in the future."

Case Study: Breast Cancer

Physician Testimony

✿ DR. DWIGHT MCKEE, M.D., ONCOLOGIST

"After practicing yoga daily for only a few months, evidence of its benefits to my own health and immune system are very apparent. My approach to cancer treatment is to integrate the very latest conventional therapies with the most promising alternative approaches."

Some lifestyle factors have been documented to be associated with an increased risk for breast cancer: obesity, alcohol, cigarettes and a high-fat diet. By helping establish a peaceful experience of body and mind, yoga practice can help people modify these risks and so help prevent breast cancer.

> Love has no boundaries; it is the greatest force on earth.
>
> —H.H. SRI SWAMI SATCHIDANANDA

In addition, wearing a bra has been found to increase the risk for breast cancer. Most likely, constriction of the breasts interferes with the body's self-regulating mechanisms to circulate nutrients and maintain healthy cells. Increased circulation resulting from yoga practice can assist the body in this self-regulation.

Once a person has developed breast cancer, yoga practice has been known to help them cope by giving them a sense of peace and tranquillity during a very stressful diagnosis and treatment. The gentle asana stretches can be particularly helpful during recovery from lumpectomy or mastectomy, to loosen the muscles in the chest, arm and shoulder affected by these procedures.

Case Study: Prostate Cancer

Increased fat in the diet is felt to be a trigger for prostate cancer. The excess fat may interfere directly with circulation or shift hormone balances to encourage tumor formation and growth.

By assisting in the maintenance of calm awareness, yoga practices may help practitioners regulate their dietary fat intake. In addition, by placing the body in the various postures of yoga, improved circulation and nutrient delivery may help the body in its self-regulatory activity for maintaining optimum cell health. This may act to help prevent prostate cancer.

Once a tumor has developed, yoga practice is known to reduce stress during this difficult time. It also helps support the immune function in its ability to fight the disease.

> *Love the moment, and the energy of that moment will spread beyond all boundaries.*
>
> —CORITA KENT, ARTIST

Case Study: Immune System Imbalances

Physician Testimony

DR. GREENFIELD, MEDICAL DIRECTOR, CAROLINAS INTEGRATIVE HEALTH CLINIC, CHARLOTTE, NORTH CAROLINA

"Health is balance. When your life is out of balance, you open the door to disharmony and disease. During a two-year fellowship with Dr. Andrew Weil at the University of Arizona, I learned that the basis of integrative medicine is a healing relationship between practitioner and patient, and the goal is to optimize the patient's 'innate healing capacity.'

"I came to integrative medicine after a decade as an ER doctor and medical director, where I often saw patients treated for physical trauma leave the hospital with 'gaping spiritual and emotional wounds.' My clinical staff, which includes an acupuncturist, herbalist, two massage therapists, a mind-body specialist, nutritionist and yoga instructor, treats the whole person. In addition to evaluating the physical symptoms and medical history, our staff works with the patient to examine their entire personal and environmental history before defining a pathway back to wellness. All modalities available at Carolinas have been proven effective by research data. We use the best of both complementary and traditional medicine to

> *Nothing will benefit the human health and increase the chances for survival of life on earth as much as evolution to the vegetarian diet.*
>
> —ALBERT EINSTEIN

promote health and well-being in the hopes that the patient will begin to rely less on the healthcare system and more on him- or herself.

"I believe that yoga is an ideal tool to promote self-care and optimize health. In the beginning I had a misperception of yoga. I like to think of myself as a jock: basketball, baseball, football always appealed to me—not yoga. But after the first class I was a convert. Our clinic offers a therapeutic yoga program that focuses on restorative postures. It is individualized and geared toward patients coping with health issues such as heart disease, cancer, lower-back pain and anxiety and depression. The whole purpose of the class is to find comfort."

> *A journey of a thousand miles must begin with a single step.*
>
> —LAOTZU

Case Study: Colon Cancer

Physician Testimony

DR. NICHOLAS PAPPAS, M.D., PSYCHIATRIST

"Ms. Buffy Stewart, a patient of mine, was quite distressed and depressed about her ongoing battle with cancer. She committed herself to regular yoga (meditation and asanas). The yoga/meditation helped her calm the turmoil within her by relaxing and better focusing her healing energies. In my opinion, her yoga practice was instrumental in her well-being today."

ROBERT F. SPETZLER, NEUROSURGEON

"It is always gratifying when patients assume responsibility for their recovery, as in the case of Ms. Buffy Stewart, and identify helpful therapeutic adjuncts after surgery. In her case yoga appears to have been an excellent vehicle to help her regain her health and well-being. Clearly the paths to healing are many, mysterious and often tinged with the miraculous."

Patient Testimony

 BUFFY FORD STEWART

"In 2001, after recovering from a benign brain tumor, I was diagnosed with colorectal cancer. This was the greatest test of my life. I was given the highest doses of chemo and radiation treatment that have ever been given. I have never been so ill or felt such harm to my body. It is said that getting chemo and radiation therapy is like setting off a nuclear bomb in your body. I really thought I was going to die. I became very depressed.

> *I always try to balance the light with the heavy—a few tears of human spirit in with the sequins and fringes.*
>
> —BETTE MIDLER

"Through all of it, I would do visualizations. I took myself to beautiful places like the ocean. I would see myself lying on the hot sand, listening to the waves, the birds, smelling the salt air. I would go through each part of my body, seeing myself totally healthy. Then I would meditate, which would bring my spirit back. It is through these yoga practices that I would realize I am not the body, not the mind, but pure spirit. I could feel God. The great love and total peace and comfort. I began to feel regenerated and my body began to gradually heal. Positive thinking and alternate nostril breathing exercises always took away my stress and fear.

> *Whenever I would dip my toes into the river of despair*
> *A mustard seed of faith would scream and would not take me there.*
> *I'll dance until I cannot breathe, until I have to crawl*
> *Until I've reached the highest peak But never will I fall.*
>
> —BUFFY STEWART

"Eventually I was able to begin doing a few yoga asanas that I had learned from guru Swami Satchidananda, like the Forward Bend, the Cobra and the Fish Pose, in my bed. Through the yoga my body continued to regenerate. I got excited and regained my faith and courage, and was inspired to return to perfect health. With the added help of acupressure treatments I received from Nirmala Heriza and the acupuncture from Dr. Samual Wang of San Rafael, California, and Dr. David Kearney from Santa Monica, California, today my health is back.

"Western medicine is just beginning to realize the power of prayer and the healing effects of yoga, known about and practiced for over three thousand years in Eastern civilizations. I am living proof that all of this is true, and it is there for everyone."

Case Study: Chronic Fatigue

Physician Testimony

DR. CRAIG BRADLEY, PLASTIC SURGEON

"I was at the top of my form as a Formula Ford champion race car driver when, during a race, I was involved in a very serious car crash. Because my car had an open cockpit, my entire body was seriously battered. Even though it was a lifelong passion, I resolved to quit racing for good.

"The intensity of the combination of speed and surgery had kept me going. Bereft of one of my usual adrenaline-charging outlets, I experienced a tension-filled turning point in my life. My fatigue became chronic and more apparent.

> *The body never lies.*
>
> —MARTHA GRAHAM

One of my friends suggested I try yoga. After a short period of practice, I discovered that the meditating left me feeling totally alert, free of disturbing thoughts—and it felt amazing to me. I felt released from stress, in a state of well-being that was a physical recognition of another way of approaching my life.

"My fatigue gradually disappeared; the yoga postures reversed the sensation of tightening and dragging my body around. Chanting allowed me to feel calm and soothed. During deep relaxation I felt as though I were leaving my body and floating free. I began using my time in yoga and meditation to release my daily challenges as a surgeon. I also began to recommend yoga to my patients before and after surgery, and witnessed significant improvements in pain relief, range of motion and time needed for recovery."

Case Study: HIV

The human immune system is impacted by both physical and emotional factors. Diet and stress have been shown to elicit changes in multiple aspects of this complex body system. Research has documented that meditation can increase the number of

T-4 cells (the immune cells that specifically fight infection) and their activity, as well as impact other aspects of immune function.

Increasingly, physicians and healthcare providers are using yoga with HIV and AIDS patients with excellent results, including improved mood, fewer infections and increased survival rates.

Physician Testimony

In the article "Effects of a Behavioral Stress-management Program on Anxiety, Mood, Self-Esteem and Cell Count in HIV-Positive Men," published in *Psychological Reports* in April 1995, Dr. D. N. Taylor reported that patients who had received twenty biweekly yoga sessions that included progressive deep relaxation and meditation had improved T-cell counts. This improvement was still in place at the one-month follow-up. Research conducted at Jefferson Medical College in Philadelphia showed that even one yoga class lowered the average cortisol levels in the blood. Cortisol levels are one measure of the body's perceived stress, and decreased levels reflect improved immune function.

> *HIV does not make people dangerous to know, so you can shake their hands and give them a hug. Heaven knows they need it.*
>
> —DIANA, PRINCESS OF WALES

Patient Testimony

One of Dr. McLanahan's patients, Sidney Paul Steed, found that yoga practice helped him deal with both the physical and the psychological stress of his HIV diagnosis. "What I notice most about yoga is that it helps me deal with my anxiety and feelings of isolation." His T-cell counts stopped plummeting and he felt courageous enough to join a support group and even began teaching some of the other members yoga.

Case Study: Cancer (Squamous-Cell Type)

Physician Testimony

✾ DR. DWIGHT MCKEE, ONCOLOGIST

"S.C., a fifty-year-old male, came to me after an enlarged lymph node on his neck had revealed on biopsy to be cancer of the squamous-cell type. In addition to conventional therapy with radiation and chemotherapy, the patient began yoga practice. He found that yoga made a significant difference, particularly in his ability to go to work. The yoga program enabled him to maintain the energy

> *The body is the temple of the spirit.*
>
> —I CORINTHIANS

needed to go to his office, which made all the difference in his quality of life. It helped immeasurably with successfully overcoming the side effects of chemotherapy and radiation, affecting his eventual recovery."

Case Study: Non-Hodgkin's Lymphoma

Nurse Practitioner's Testimony

✾ DEBRA MULNICK, R.N.

"Alice, a female patient of mine in her early fifties, was diagnosed with non-Hodgkin's lymphoma in 1996. She had her first chemotherapy in 2000 in an attempt to reduce the swelling of her abdominal lymph nodes, which were causing nerve pain and lymphedema of the left leg. She wore a thigh-high support stocking to help reduce leg swelling. She also reported depression as a health concern. She said she had been extremely active in the past, and a major stress factor for her was her loss of vitality. Her expectations of yoga class were that it would provide her with re-laxation and increased mobility.

"Alice attended class regularly, even on weeks when she was receiving chemotherapy and wasn't feeling very energetic. She said, 'I look forward to these classes so much. Even while I'm getting chemo, I think of yoga class as a reward at the end of the day, and it always leaves me feeling better than when I came.' The first classes emphasized a tuning-in process to help Alice become more aware of ways the body holds tension, together with breathing practices to help steady the mind.

"I slowly introduced restorative yoga poses, which use blankets and bolsters to support the body in various positions. Restorative poses give the patient an experience of very comfortable deep relaxation. One of the beneficial poses for Alice during that time was a passive supported inversion called 'elevated-legs-up-the-wall pose.' She practiced the pose with a bolster under her hips to help promote lymph drainage from the lower half of her body. I encouraged her to practice this pose regularly, as she had been complaining of her abdomen 'feeling bloated.' This pose allows one to experience a sense of spaciousness and relaxation in the belly.

"As Alice responded to chemotherapy, her abdominal node enlargement and leg swelling decreased. We slowly introduced a full range of active poses as her energy level increased. She said how much she enjoyed practicing standing poses, since she had always been a very physically active person. These poses made her feel stronger.

"Over the years Alice's treatments and health status have had many ups and downs. Sometimes her yoga consists of breathing practices only. Like many people, Alice finds alternate nostril breathing very calming. At other times she has been able to join group classes during a more strenuous practice. The most important thing is to allow her needs at the time to dictate what kind of yoga practice will best serve her on a particular day.

"She has told me, 'Yoga practice has served as a nurturing anchor as I go through the ups and downs of treatment.' She is a committed student in class and continues to practice on her own."

Nervous System/Brain

The nervous system includes the sympathetic nervous system, the parasympathetic nervous system, the autonomic nervous system, the somatic nervous system and the central nervous system. The sympathetic system controls activity and stress. It emerges from the mid back and causes the "fight or flight" response. The parasympathetic nervous system is located in the neck and lower back and produces a relaxation response. It reacts in a complementary way to the sympathetic nervous system.

The health of every tissue in the body depends on this system because nerves from the brain and spine go to all the organs and glands of the body. A healthy spine plays a vital role in vitality and rejuvenation.

The somatic nervous system contains both afferent (incoming) and efferent (outgoing) nerves. It receives and processes information passed to it by receptors in the skin, voluntary muscles, tendons, joints, eyes, tongue, nose and ears, giving us the sensations of touch, pain, heat, cold, balance, sight, taste, smell and hearing. It allows us to move our arms and legs.

CENTRAL NERVOUS SYSTEM

Brain

Spinal cord

Autonomic Nervous System

Relates to the function of the internal organs

Sympathetic Nervous System

Controls the "fight or flight" response

Parasympathetic Nervous System

Relaxation response

Somatic Nervous System

Muscular system and external sensory receptors

Disease conditions commonly related to the
autonomic and somatic nervous systems

Shingles

Migraines

Substance abuse

Insomnia

ADD (Attention Deficit Disorder)

Anxiety disorders

Fibromyalgia (Chronic fatigue)

Parkinson's disease

Meningitis

Alzheimer's disease

Epilepsy
Encephalitis
Memory loss
Stroke
Schizophrenia

The Hatha yoga asanas in the Yoga for Health restorative program have proven effective in helping to rebalance and restore the health of all of these systems.

Recommended Asanas

JANUSIRASANA (HEAD-TO-KNEE POSE)

Massages the parasympathetic nervous system (nerves situated in the lower spine), producing a relaxation effect helpful in the management of anxiety and stress. See page 99.

SARVANGASANA (SHOULDERSTAND)

(To be done either supported or unsupported)

Particularly strategic to the support of the sympathetic and parasympathetic nervous systems, which make up the autonomic nervous system. In addition, by increasing blood flow to the scalp and brain, this pose has been clinically observed to promote vitality and increase memory and IQ. Nerves from the brain go to every tissue of the body. Therefore, the body is dependent on the health of the brain and spine. See pages 102–104.

❀ MATSYASANA (FISH POSE) ❀

Extends the muscles of the neck, shoulders and back, helping to increase the space between vertebrae, allowing them to breathe and alleviating any stress in the area. It also increases circulation to the brain stem and the cranial nerves. It should always follow the Shoulderstand. See page 104.

❀ YOGA NIDRA (DEEP RELAXATION) ❀

The body and mind are interconnected and interdependent. The body expresses the thoughts of the mind. If you have a happy mind, your face and body will reflect that happiness.

—H.H. Sri Swami Satchidananda

Simply by progressively releasing tension from each part of the body and increasing circulation by contracting and releasing the muscles, yoga nidra helps restore the natural health of the body's entire nervous system. Lying in the supine position, all of the nerves and vertebrae that support the spine are allowed to "let go" and completely relax, helping to promote normal spinal alignment. I have used this practice with my private patients as an adjunct treatment for migraine headache, in many cases clinically noted to be caused by stress and poor circulation. See page 109.

❀ KAPALA BATHI (SKULL SHINING) ❀

You're only given a little spark of madness. You mustn't lose it.

—Robin Williams

Because of the "vitality" and "energy" produced by the vigorous repetition of breaths in this pose, the entire nervous system is revitalized and strengthened. See page 28.

NADDI SUDDHI (ALTERNATE NOSTRIL BREATHING)

By relaxing, purifying and strengthening the subtle nerve currents along the spine and in the brain, alternate nostril breathing helps prevent memory loss and restore memory as well as reduce mental and emotional stress. It is strategically effective in diffusing the effects of negative emotions such as anger, fear and anxiety, as well as helping to lift depression. See page 111.

> *Worry gives a small thing a big shadow.*
> —Swedish proverb

Case Study: Depression

As many as 25 million Americans take antidepressants regularly. Unfortunately, these medications are often accompanied by significant side effects such as fatigue, weight gain, tremors, sleep disturbance and loss of sexual functioning. Yoga practice has been documented to help alleviate depression, and the programs in this book may be utilized to help prevent and treat this prevalent disorder.

According to Dr. Mehmet Oz of New York Presbyterian Hospital's cardiology department, people who experience depression are at four times the risk of suffering a heart attack and are less likely to survive open-heart surgery. The heart-lung machine utilized during such heart procedures, in addition to depressing the immune system, is associated with inducing higher rates of psychological depression postoperatively. Dr. Oz recommends yoga to patients before and after surgery to help reduce the risk of depression.

> *I get by with a little help from my friends.*
> —John Lennon

Dr. S. Khumar and associates published an article entitled "Effectiveness of Savasana on Depression Among University Students" in the *Indian Journal of Clinical Psychology* (vol. 20, 1993). In their controlled study they found that fifty university students diagnosed with severe depression were signficiantly relieved of their depressive symptoms when given thirty sessions of deep relaxation.

Physician Testimony

Dr. James Gordon, director of the Center for Mind-Body Medicine in Washington, D.C., is a clinical psychiatrist who has worked at the National Institutes of Mental Health. He recognizes yoga and meditation as modalities for the treatment of stress and anxiety disorders. He also served as chairman of the White House Commission on Complementary Medicine Policy in 2002. In the November 14, 2000, issue of *The Washington Post,* he stated: "A new kind of medicine is developing in this country that sees patients as fellow human beings and looks to other healing traditions."

> *The claims of habit are generally too small to be felt until they are too strong to be broken.*
>
> —SAMUEL JOHNSON, STATESMAN

Patient Testimony

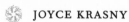 **JOYCE KRASNY**

"At the time that I was diagnosed by my physician, Hark Nachman, M.D., with hypertension, I began experiencing depression and fear of dying or being incapacitated by a stroke. I was taking medication to control the symptoms. At the suggestion of both my primary physician and a psychotherapist, I began doing yoga for my condition in 2001 with Leslie Bogart, who is both a registered nurse and a certified yoga instructor.

"At first I was reluctant to try yoga because I was skeptical that it could help me. I was also resistant to the group setting of the class. Because of that alone I was sure I would hate it. However, after giving it a try for a few weeks I found it helped me to relax. I also credit Ms. Bogart, who is well versed in physical disease, for providing individualized quality attention to each member of the class and for making it a valuable experience.

> *Cocaine isn't habit forming. I should know. I've been using it for years.*
>
> —TALLULAH BANKHEAD, ACTRESS

"Although I continue to suffer from labile hypertension, my physician has told me that my overall health has improved. My yoga therapist, in particular, is very enthusiastic about the quality of my mental health and my ability to relax, critical to my A-type personality."

Case Study: Substance Abuse

In research conducted at Harvard, Dr. Herbert Benson found that meditation and the subsequent decrease in stress levels are effective in helping patients free themselves of abusive substances. The results of his research were published in 1975 in the *International Journal of Psychiatry and Medicine,* "The Relaxation Response: Psychological Aspects and Clinical Applications."

> *There are three side effects of acid. Enhanced long-term memory, decreased short-term memory, and I forget the rest.*
>
> —TIMOTHY LEARY

Physician Testimony

 DR. HERBERT BENSON, M.D.

"Yoga has been shown to be very effective in reducing stress and strengthening the body. Now we are looking at how the practice can enhance wellness in a population beset by health problems. Asana and pranayama are specifically selected to enhance relaxation and facilitate healing." Further significant risks in the onset of stress-related "seizures" have been determined through significant clinical studies by Dr. U. Panjawani of the Defense Institute of Physiology and Allied Sciences in New Delhi, India, published in the *Indian Journal of Medical Research* in 1996. After three months of yoga training, the chronic-seizure disorder patients in the control study exhibited a 62 percent reduction in seizures. After six months, an 86 percent reduction was seen.

> *The sensible man will just light a candle and bring it into the room. Yoga is that candle. Bring it into your life and all your unwanted habits will leave. You need not bother yourself about them. When the mind and body are strong, they will just drop away.*
>
> —H.H. SRI SWAMI SATCHIDANANDA

Case Study: Bipolar Disorder

Bipolar disorder is a psychiatric illness characterized by fluctuations between anxiety and depression. Yoga practice can be a useful adjunct to conventional medical treatment and in some cases may enable patients to free themselves of medication altogether, although this must be accomplished only with close medical supervision.

Yoga increases serotonin levels in the brain, which can help alleviate both anxiety and depression. Serotonin, a hormone produced by the neurons, is associated with tranquillity. In addition, by balancing the sympathetic (alertness) and parasympathetic (relaxation) portions of the nervous system, yoga practice can help during the continuing cycle of manic and depressed phases of this disorder. Daily practice is essential, especially emphasizing alternate nostril breathing, which acts quickly to calm, uplift and stabilize the mind.

> *See, the human mind is kind of like a piñata. When it breaks open, there's a lot of surprises inside. Once you get the piñata perspective, you see that losing your mind can be a peak experience.*
>
> —JANE WAGNER, WRITER

Patient Testimony

 C.S.

C.S., a thirty-eight-year-old male, had suffered from bipolar disorder since childhood. Despite medication, he was experiencing significant mood swings that were interfering with his work. After adding yoga practice to his life, he reported that he felt truly free of depression for the first time. He was also able to reduce his psychoactive medication, which he greatly appreciated as it had been causing significant unwanted side effects.

> *We shall find peace. We shall hear the angels, we shall see the sky sparkling with diamonds.*
>
> —ANTON CHEKHOV, 1897

Case Study: Epilepsy

Physician Testimony

 DR. STEPHEN PACIA

The NYU Comprehensive Epilepsy Center offers yoga to patients. Preliminary studies indicate that an alternative therapy such as yoga may be used effectively in reducing stress and seizures in patients with epilepsy. The proven benefits of yoga have led to its inclusion as an integral component in the medical management of numerous disorders. Dr. Pacia is studying yoga as a means of reducing seizure frequency and improving anxiety and depression. While studies are ongoing, Dr. Pacia says the staff receives positive feedback from nearly all participants. Instructors tailor classes to the abilities of each patient, and even patients who have never exercised enjoy yoga. He states that "the program focuses on reducing seizure frequency, maximizing rehabilitation and improving quality of life." A gentle form of yoga is taught that does not involve strenuous movement. The classes are structured so that the last half hour is devoted to breathing exercises and meditation.

> *I am but mad north-northwest: when the wind is southerly I know a hawk from a handsaw.*
>
> —WILLIAM SHAKESPEARE

NYU's Comprehensive Epilepsy Center is the largest epilepsy program in the eastern United States. It offers testing, evaluation, screening, medical and surgical treatment, clinical drug tests and alternative therapies to children, adolescents, and adults with all forms of epilepsy, through inpatient and outpatient programs.

Patient Testimony

 JOE

"I'm a professional actor who began taking part in the Yoga Research Project at NYU Epilepsy Center about two and a half years ago. At that time, I was experiencing two or three seizures over a six-month period, even though I was taking medication (Dilantin, 400 mg per day).

"I didn't notice much difference at first, except for an increasing awareness of different parts of my body, those parts we take for granted because we don't use them much. And I became aware of muscular tensions that were caused by my emotional anxieties.

> *Discipline makes your mind stronger and one-pointed. It should ultimately help you make your mind your slave. Don't be controlled by anything. Exercise your Mastery. That is the aim of Yoga.*
>
> —H.H. SRI SWAMI SATCHIDANANDA

"The practice helped me identify and release tensions that in the past would build up until they were released by a seizure. I had one seizure about two months after beginning the practice, and then went for nearly a year, until one was triggered by a personal family difficulty. I have now gone eight months without a seizure.

"Because I had epileptic seizures, I finally gave up trying to work as an actor. The behind-the-scenes pressures and anxieties involved were just too much for me; or rather, I allowed them to become too much because I had no tool with which to control them. That is what yoga has become for me. Now I am singing, which was my first love, and trying to put a cabaret act together. Should the opportunity arise, I would definitely try acting again. I take yoga instruction twice a week at NYU Medical Center, and practice forty-five minutes to an hour at home on other days. As my instructor confirmed, I believe that doing it on a daily basis is more beneficial than just doing it once or twice a week. You actually receive from it what you put into it. It's like buying *The New York Times*—you must read it to be informed. Just buying it isn't enough."

> *Many people don't think it's fashionable to sneeze or cough. Don't let "civilized" habits stop the body's natural elimination. You cause great damage to the body and affect hundreds of nerves by controlling your sneezing and coughing. When you sneeze, God will bless you.*
>
> —H.H. Sri Swami Satchidananda

Respiratory System

Recommended Asanas

✿ BHUJANGASANA (COBRA POSE) ✿

Stimulates the thyroid gland at the base of throat, helping to stabilize the metabolism and lower blood cholesterol. The back muscles are strengthened. The spine becomes more supple and the chest expands, promoting oxygen and circulation to the lungs and heart. See page 97.

✿ MATSYASANA (FISH POSE) ✿

Increases circulation into the lungs and heart. As reported in the *Journal of the American Medical Association* (*JAMA*), the Fish Pose is clinically recognized as effective in treating asthma and bronchial conditions. See page 104.

KAPALA BATHI (SKULL SHINING)

Brings heat to the body when it's cold. Improves digestion, removes phlegm and helps in the prevention and treatment of asthma and other respiratory diseases. It exhilarates the blood circulation and energizes the entire body quickly. See page 28.

Case Study: Asthma

In its September 2003 *Health Letter,* the Mayo Clinic reported that yoga breathing techniques (*pranayama*) are an effective clinical strategy for nourishing the blood, cleansing waste products from the lungs and reducing stress. The clinic recommends the practice of deep, rhythmic breathing techniques to increase the volume of oxygen in the lungs, strengthen the respiratory system and reduce stress. It encourages developing the habit of breathing through the nose, not the mouth, to filter out toxins and calm the nervous system.

> *That you exceed not the bounds, but observe the balance strictly, and fall not short thereof.*
>
> —QURAN (55-7-9)

In terms of clinical benefit, the Mayo Clinic suggests there is evidence that yoga practices (physical postures and breathing techniques) can be effective in the treatment of asthma as well as heart disease, cancer, chemical dependence, anxiety-related disorders and depression. In summary, this world-renowned and respected medical institution has given yoga its strong endorsement for both prevention and treatment of various acute and chronic diseases.

> *The best nutrition can be no better than the condition of your colon. When your colon is clogged, your nutrients do not absorb efficiently.*
>
> —Dr. Bernard Jensen

Physician Testimony

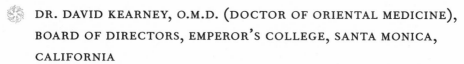 DR. DAVID KEARNEY, O.M.D. (DOCTOR OF ORIENTAL MEDICINE), BOARD OF DIRECTORS, EMPEROR'S COLLEGE, SANTA MONICA, CALIFORNIA

"Asthmatics traditionally gulp in too much air. For many decades it has been recognized by the medical community that hyperventilation occurs in asthmatics. Asthmatics can take in up to three times their normal required breath. Because we live in a world that thinks more oxygen and more food is better, obesity and asthma, along with other related acute and chronic conditions, are all too common.

"When an asthmatic sucks in air quickly through the mouth, they become more susceptible to a wide range of conditions, including respiratory, nervous and immune disorders and even muscle and joint tension. When a person hyperventilates, it interferes with the healthy balance of oxygen and carbon dioxide. This oxygen-rich condition tips the balance between the body's oxygen and carbon dioxide levels. This results in a more acidic pH, a condition commonly found in asthma patients.

> *The best remedy for any illness is laughter.*
>
> —H.H. Sri Swami Satchidananda

"Human beings are creatures of routine. Breathing correctly is the best habit you can give yourself. By conditioning your body toward slow, nasal, deep, rhythmic breathing, exemplified in Hatha yoga, rhythmic breath becomes a very healthy physiological habit. This leads to overall balance, more energy and a way to truly tap into your healing power."

Gastrointestinal System

Recommended Asanas

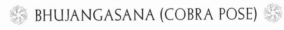 BHUJANGASANA (COBRA POSE)

Provides a gentle massage to the abdomen. According to clinical studies, this pose creates an increase in pressure within the stomach (measured in millimeters of mercury, it produces the equivalent of 40 to 50 mm of mercury). The kidneys and adrenal glands are also massaged, improving circulation and helping to prevent stone formation. See page 97.

JANUSIRASANA (HEAD-TO-KNEE POSE)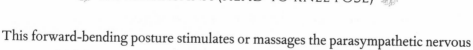

This forward-bending posture stimulates or massages the parasympathetic nervous system, which has nerves in the lower spine. The massage of these fibers produces a relaxation effect that feels good. Systemically, it promotes circulation to the lower bowel, helping to prevent constipation and hemorrhoids. The increased blood supply can help the body repair the muscles and lining of the bowel, while the gentle pressure facilitates movement of food along the digestive tract. Since it directly stimulates the parasympathetic nervous system, it causes the contents of the bowel to move along more effectively. See page 99.

PASCHIMOTHANASANA (FULL FORWARD BEND)

Stimulates, massages and relaxes the pelvic floor muscles. See page 101.

SARVANGASANA (SHOULDERSTAND)

Regular practice of the Shoulderstand can provide both a preventive measure and relief from hemorrhoids, which result when the constant pressure of gravity exceeds what the valves in the veins can handle. See pages 102–104.

> Too much of a good thing is wonderful.
> —Mae West

CAVEAT: If your condition is acute or you are recovering from surgery, do the modified version of this pose. Always consult with your phsycian before attempting the pose.

ARDDHAMATSYANDRASANA (HALF SPINAL TWIST)

Provides a twisting action that engages the entire length of the spine. The middle part of the body, at the level of the kidneys and adrenals, benefits particularly. Increased pressure in the stomach of 30 to 40 mm of mercury has been measured. See page 106.

YOGA MUDRA (YOGIC SEAL)

Referred to in H.H. Sri Swami Satchidananda's *Integral Yoga Hatha* as "the symbol of Yoga," this is considered a very powerful pose that should finish any session of postures. It stimulates the parasympathetic nervous system and increases stomach pressure by 20 mm of mercury. The heels contact the lower bowel, massaging it and helping to prevent or alleviate constipation. See page 108.

❀ DEERGA SWASAM (DEEP BREATHING) ❀

Relaxes the muscles in the lower back that support the abdominal region, as well as the abdominal muscles and viscera, by increasing circulation into those areas, thereby helping to alleviate abdominal stress and discomfort. See page 111.

❀ KAPALA BATHI (SKULL SHINING) ❀

This breathing technique massages the abdominal organs, helping to prevent constipation and other abdominal complaints. See page 28.

❀ NADDI SUDDHI (ALTERNATE NOSTRIL BREATHING) ❀

Promotes good appetite and proper digestion. See page 111.

Case Study: Irritable Bowel Syndrome

Physician Testimony

 DR. RICHARD PANICO, M.D., CHIEF OF PSYCHIATRY AND
MEDICAL DIRECTOR OF THE MIND-BODY INSTITUTE OF THE
ATHENS, GEORGIA, REGIONAL MEDICAL CENTER HOSPITAL

"By age forty I was completely exhausted from the demands of my private psychiatry practice; my problem progressed beyond mere simple tiredness. In addition to debilitating fatigue, I developed a severe viral infection with irritable bowel syndrome, cardiomyopathy, hepatitis and hypertension. My own doctor advised me to cash in on my disability and retire early.

> *Who is the man who enjoys food? The one who eats well, chews well, digests well and assimilates well; not the one who eats for the sake of his tongue, overloads his stomach, and then uses purgatives.*
>
> —H.H. Sri Swami Satchidananda

"However, I love my work and thought I was too young to retire, so I decided to try an alternative approach. I remembered that when I was in college, where I was first exposed to and began practicing yoga, my grades improved and I could do my 'iron cross' gymnastics position more effectively. At the time it didn't occur to me that my yoga routine was actually making such a difference. Since I didn't really make the association and value it, I left it behind once I entered medical school.

"I thought perhaps I should give it a try again, just to see if it might somehow benefit me. Unlike exercise, I found that yoga classes didn't leave me feeling more tired; instead I felt energized. Having researched the profound effects that yoga can have on the body's cellular metabolism, I found that when the body profoundly relaxes as a result of the yoga, it says, in effect, 'No stress here, you can do repair work.'

> *Half the game is 90 percent mental.*
>
> —Yogi Berra

"As a result of my practice, my heart and liver function tests began to improve, and I turned the corner on my disease and all of its related conditions. Having experienced such subjective and objective improvement in my own health with yoga, I founded clinics at my medical center, the Athens Regional Medical Center in Augusta, Georgia, to teach and research the application of yoga for patients suffering from chronic pain, migraines, chronic back pain, headaches and other chronic and stress-related disorders. My patients have demonstrated such remarkable progress that other staff physicians are now eagerly referring their patients to these clinics for yoga treatment."

Professional Health Practitioner's Testimony

NIRMALA HERIZA, B.A., CYT

"D.L., a film actor, producer and writer, is a middle-aged female private patient of mine who presented with the diagnosis of an irritable bowel condition for which she was hospitalized. The day after being discharged she began seeing me for acupressure and Hatha yoga therapy. She was experiencing bloating and cramping in the lower abdominal area with associated diarrhea. She was limited to eating broth and drinking fluids, and complained that solid food irritated her stomach.

"At first I had her do deep relaxation and the pranayama practices until her strength returned. Gradually, after one week, her energy began to return, and I had her begin doing the posterior (forward-bending) poses recommended in this book. I also suggested she consult with a nutrition specialist for dietary recommendations.

"After three weeks, when she was able to begin resuming her normal daily activities, I recommended she begin doing the full thirty-minute Yoga for Health restorative program (Practice Set II) once a week along with her modified program. Today she has fully regained her health. She experiences only occasional exacerbations of her condition when her Hatha yoga practice lapses."

> *A wise man should consider that health is the greatest of human blessings—and learn how by his own thought to derive benefit from his illness.*
>
> —HIPPOCRATES

USING VISUALIZATION TECHNIQUES TO COMPLEMENT YOUR HATHA YOGA PRACTICE

Whether you are rehabilitating after surgery, undergoing postoperative therapy such as chemotherapy or radiation or paralyzed and unable to move, for patients who are restricted in their movement or confined to a bed, visualizing the Hatha yoga asanas has been proven to be an effective method of treatment. The mind is a powerful instrument and, combined with the breathing techniques, visualization is known to be almost as effective as physically doing the postures.

Mentally picture yourself doing each asana as if you were participating in a routine class. Do the yoga nidra (deep relaxation) component as usual. If necessary, imagine yourself tensing and releasing each body part. If you have mobility of your upper extremities, you can do the pranayama practices as usual. If you don't, you can at least do the deep breathing, and even picture yourself doing Naddi Suddhi (alternative nostril breathing) along with your deep breathing.

Guided Visualization

When Dr. Ornish first began developing his program for reversing heart disease, he contacted his guru, Swami Satchidananda, to ask for any recommendations and guidance he might have for cardiac patients in addition to Hatha yoga, pranayama (breathing) practices and meditation techniques.

> *There is nothing either good or bad but thinking makes it so.*
>
> —Shakespeare, *Hamlet* II:ii

Swami Satchidananda suggested that his patients use guided imagery or visualization to help promote the healing experience. For patients with blocked coronary arteries, for example, he suggested they imagine a Roto-Rooter device tunneling through the blockages, cleaning and opening up the arteries. He also advised Dr. Ornish to encourage patients to use their imagination in the technique.

In his research into the effects of visualization techniques, Dr. Ornish cited a study in which psychologist Richard Suinn, Ph.D., recorded muscle activity in a skier while he visualized himself racing downhill. The measured readings were similar to those made when someone was actually skiing downhill.

Other studies have demonstrated that visualizing terrible things happening decreases blood flow to the heart. Conversely, visualizing positive images improves coronary blood flow by dilating the coronary arteries to some degree. According to Dr. Ornish, there is evidence suggesting that visualization may reduce the number and severity of irregular heartbeats. More specific information on the relationship between visualization and coronary artery disease and how to apply the practice to this condition is outlined in detail in Ornish's best-selling book *Program for Reversing Heart Disease*.

> *As you think, so you become. Think well, you will be well. Think ill, you will be ill. It's all your thought.*
>
> —H.H. Sri Swami Satchidananda

The same visualization principles can be applied to any condition. There are many excellent books available on the practice of visualization and guided imagery. Some are listed in the reference section at the back of this book.

Clinical Testimony

🌀 **NIRMALA HERIZA, B.A., CYT**

"M.'s case is a compelling example of how visualization techniques can be a powerful adjunct to therapy. M. was scheduled for a heart transplant. Because it is such a radical procedure, his physician at Cedars-Sinai Medical Center suggested that he consult with Dr. Ornish to see if he could suggest a clinical alternative. After reviewing M.'s case and talking with him, Dr. Ornish convinced him to wait on the surgery and first try yoga therapy and a low-fat vegetarian nutritional regime. If that didn't improve his symptoms, there would still be time to go ahead with the surgery.

> *Peace is your nature. It is who you really are—while everything else is a distraction. The mind gets pulled into worries and concerns, it gets drawn away from its true source that is internal, it becomes deluded and identified with external phenomena. Soon you are caught up in the drama and chaos.*
>
> —*UNCONDITIONAL LOVE*, ED AND DEBBIE SHAPIRO

"Dr. Ornish referred the patient to me and I began supervising him in the modified Integral Yoga–based cardiac program six days a week. In addition to following the diet and doing the yoga and relaxation practices, M. was also implementing the visualization techniques that Dr. Ornish had advised him to do. A creative person, M. improvised a unique way of looking at his heart that inspired his healing process. He envisioned his heart filled with a bright gold and purple light.

"Each day I encouraged him to relate to me in detail how his heart appeared during the visualizations and how he felt. Initially, he was very depressed, enervated by his condition and frightened by the ultimate possibility of having to undergo a traumatic heart transplant in order to live.

"Gradually, through the therapy he began to grow stronger. On one occasion, he told me he had given his heart an alter ego: that of a warrior overcoming a giant disease in the form of a mountain that had invaded his heart. In his visualizations he would chip away at the mountain with an iron pike. He also began drawing the image of his heart affected by the disease on a sketch pad, and was surprised to see how gradually he was inspired to draw it looking healthier.

"As he continued to experience his strength returning, he related to me that he no longer had to create a mental picture of his heart and its alter ego; the image became spontaneous. As the warrior got stronger, the obstacle began to diminish in size. It began to appear automatically in his meditation and during the yoga relaxation.

"After just three weeks of diligent therapy, using only the relaxation and visualization techniques and the Ornish diet, M.'s blood pressure and other clinical statistics began to stabilize. After two months of continued therapy he was able to begin resuming his normal daily activities. His primary physician at Cedars-Sinai Medical Center was astounded by the speed and effectiveness of his recovery.

> *For us physicists, the distinction between past, present and future is only an illusion.*
>
> —ALBERT EINSTEIN

"M. believes that the visualization was a significant contributing factor in his ability to overcome the debilitating depression and fatigue that were components of his heart disease."

Physician Testimony

Dr. Sandra McLanahan, a strong exponent of visualization, relates that one of her patients, Grace Wilson, had developed a serious heart inflammation, called myocarditis. For six months she lay languishing in bed, unable to walk more than a few steps without becoming short of breath. Dr. McLanahan suggested that she try visualizing her heart muscle getting stronger, and brought in a bulb syringe and some water to better help her "see" this happen-

> *Meditation is not the means to an end. It is both the means and the end.*
>
> —JIDDU KRISHNAMURTHI

ing. Within two weeks of beginning her visualization practice, the fluid around her heart had reduced by 50 percent, and she felt healthy enough to play tennis.

Patient Testimony

SARASWATI NEUMANN, RECOVERED CANCER PATIENT

"Cancer is an immune system problem. It is our own cells that have mutated and do not know that they are supposed to stop growing. They continue to grow and invade the surrounding tissue. They don't know when to stop. I spoke to them and said, 'Hey, guys. Don't you know if you keep this up the body will die and then I will find another place to live and you will find yourself with no home, buried under a big pile of dirt?' I think they got the message. I also found that hoping for the best and accepting what is and what comes is what worked for me."

Meditation

I have provided step-by-step instruction on how to meditate elsewhere in this book. For more in-depth and theoretical instruction, I recommend Swami Satchidananda's *To Know Your Self* or his guided meditation CD or audiocassette, referenced in the resource section and available in our patients' resource library at Cedars-Sinai Medical Center.

Whether you're in good health or have a serious medical condition, physically active or confined to a bed, you can follow the simple methods outlined on pages 24–26 and experience the profound effects they can have on both mind and body.

What I talk about and highlight in this section are the specific ways that meditation is being recognized and implemented by distinguished physicians, scientists and various institutions in the mainstream medical community throughout the world today. Boston cardiologist Dr. Herbert Benson and his colleague Dr. Robert Keith Wallace were the first to report a major breakthrough in the effects of meditation on the cardiovascular system. In a study conducted with students of transcendental meditation in 1968, they found that their subjects showed decreased metabolism and heart and respiratory rates while practicing "mantra" meditation. It was the opposite reaction to what is commonly referred to as the "flight-or-fight response" in a stress-induced situation.

I no longer have the fear of being alone. It's cool to find out that you don't need a boyfriend to be happy.

—DREW BARRYMORE

According to Dr. Benson, meditation "gives us the capacity to put stress back in the box." According to Dr. Ornish, Benson's research also demonstrates that meditation can improve productivity and decrease healthcare costs.

In a recent study sponsored by the National Institutes of Health, the TM (Transcendental Meditation) organization conducted a clinical trial in collaboration with Cedars-Sinai Medical Center under the supervision of Dr. C. Noel Bairey Merz, M.D., director of the Preventive and Rehabilitative Cardiac Program. The study involved middle-aged participants with no meditation experience. The results were positive. According to Dr. Merz, "when people learn how to meditate and are able to do it daily, it is an effective stress-management technique."

Handling stress is an important hurdle for patients suffering from heart-related disorders. Without significant lifestyle changes such as better nutrition, exercise and the adoption of a practice such as meditation, it is difficult to recover completely because standard procedures such as open-heart surgery, angioplasty and medication treat only the symptoms; they do not shift the patient's ability to manage tension and develop a sense of wellness.

> *The cosmic religious experience is the strongest and noblest driving force behind scientific research.*
>
> —ALBERT EINSTEIN

Other studies conducted by the TM group produced impressive findings that demonstrate the effectiveness of meditation in reducing the risk of heart attack, stroke and atherosclerosis. Reductions among the meditators were comparable to those using medication and lifestyle modifications.

As I mentioned earlier, it is due to Swami Satchidananda's influence and under his direct guidance that Dr. Ornish, as a medical student at Harvard, first began researching meditation as a mechanism for treating heart disease. The depth of his scientific exploration led him to observe that the physiological effects of meditation, such as lowering blood pressure and even helping to reverse heart disease, are only side effects or by-products of its primary purpose: the experience of inner peace, happiness and oneness, which begins to heal our isolation. The feeling of isolation, as Swami Satchidananda teaches, and as Dr. Ornish's further research has revealed, is a significant factor in developing not only heart disease but disease in general. Whether we choose to believe it or not, as a part of the entire creation we are all interconnected. We're one common life force in different shapes and sizes.

As Einstein so eloquently put it, "A human being is a part of a whole, called by us ... universe ... a part limited in time and space. He experiences himself, his thoughts and feelings as something separated from the rest ... a kind of optical delusion of his consciousness. . . . This delusion is a kind of prison for us, restricting us to our personal desires and to affection for a few persons nearest to us. Our task must be to free ourselves from this prison by widening our circle of compassion to embrace all living creatures and the whole of nature in its beauty."

Swami Satchidananda teaches that one of the fundamental principles of yoga is "unity in diversity," which, he also notes, is an underlying theory of quantum physics. We are each one of us a part of the essential energy that makes up and sustains the entire universe. As Dr. Ornish observes, "Through Einstein's equation on relativity, $e = mc^2$ (energy equals mass times the speed of light squared), he demonstrates that energy and matter are incontrovertible. In other words, everything in the universe is a manifestation of different forms of energy. The forms change; the underlying essence does not."

This is where science and what Einstein refers to as "cosmic religion" converge. By recognizing the underlying scientific theories that are fundamental in meditation and yoga, the medical community is beginning to help bridge the two worlds.

PART
Three

Nutrition

by Mary Felando, M.S., R.D.,
Cardiovascular Nutrition Specialist for the
Preventive and Rehabilitative Cardiac Center
at Cedars-Sinai Medical Center

Yoga-Friendly Foods

Introduction: Sample a Refreshing Change of Taste!

The American diet is characterized by excessive amounts of saturated fat, cholesterol and calories and inadequate amounts of fruits, vegetables and fiber. For the average American, 34 percent of daily calories come from fat, with a whopping 12 percent in the form of saturated artery-clogging fat. A jump in calorie intake due to ever-increasing portion sizes has led, in part, to an obesity epidemic in our country. With fruit and vegetable intake below par, at 3 to 4 servings per day, it isn't surprising that we also fall short of our fiber target! Research has shown that our unhealthful diet is linked to high rates of heart disease, obesity, high blood pressure, stroke, diabetes and cancer. Isn't it time we take a good long look at our eating habits and make a change for the better?

The Yoga-Friendly Foods Plan focuses on health-enhancing, plant-based foods that can be conveniently purchased and simply prepared as part of your active and busy lifestyle. This style of eating is one that we use at the Preventive and Rehabilitative Cardiac Center at Cedars-Sinai Medical Center. We believe this eating plan has been instrumental in the recovery of many of our patients. We also use it to prevent heart disease and keep our patients healthy!

Keep an open mind as you read about the foods that will improve your health and well-being. Try making food choices that take you in the *direction* of a healthier eating style. No one is perfect! The move toward healthier eating is a journey with ups and downs. Expect that there will be "downs" and use them as opportunities for growth. As you begin to feel more energetic and directed, you will find that you actually enjoy your new eating style!

The Yoga-Friendly Foods Plan is a lacto-ovo vegetarian eating plan. It is derived from a blend of goals set forth by the Adult Treatment Panel III of the National Cholesterol Education Program, the American Heart Association Dietary Guidelines 2000, the Dietary Approaches to Stop Hypertension (DASH), the American Institute for Cancer Research, the Lifestyle Heart Trial, the Lyon Diet Heart Study and the author's twenty years of experience as a cardiovascular nutritionist.

NUTRITIONAL CHARACTERISTICS OF THE YOGA-FRIENDLY FOODS PLAN
- plant-based
- eliminates all animal flesh
- allows eggs and dairy
- 20–30% of calories from fat
- fewer than 7% of calories from saturated fat
- less than 100 mg cholesterol per day
- at least 25 grams fiber per day
- calories to maintain or achieve a healthier weight

FOODS TO INCLUDE
- 10 servings of fruits and vegetables per day
- 2–4 servings of protein-rich foods per day (emphasis on beans and soy)
- 2–3 servings of non-fat/low-fat dairy or soy alternative per day
- fats and oils—primarily unsaturated and including nuts
- whole grains
- moderate intake of sugar, salt and alcohol

NOTE: The nutritional plan I have laid out here allows you to eat eggs and to drink moderate amounts of alcohol. However, the Integral Yoga teachings of Sri Swami Satchidananda on which Nirmala Heriza based the theoretical and instructional portion of this book advocate a more literal interpretation of vegetarianism. While Integral Yoga dietary guidelines permit dairy, they do not permit eggs. Additionally, Nirmala Heriza explains that alcohol can disturb the systemic balance of mind and body necessary for the practice of yoga and meditation. For more information on the physiological and ethical rationale underlying this more orthodox vegetarian and dietary philosophy, please refer to Swami Satchidananda's *The Healthy Vegetarian*, listed in the resource directory.

If this eating plan is far from your usual, don't be discouraged. In my practice at Cedars-Sinai Medical Center I've met with thousands of individuals who felt, like you perhaps, that a meal was not complete without beef or poultry. If they ate any vegetables, it was a pickle with a pastrami sandwich or an iceberg lettuce salad loaded with fatty dressing. Many have successfully made the switch to more plant-based eating. Some were very motivated by a recent cardiac event (heart attack, angioplasty or bypass operation). One man expressed it aptly: "There's nothing like a heart attack to help you change your life! I never want to feel that scared again!" If the prospect of eating fleshless meals with ten fruits and veggies and beans and non-fat dairy is overwhelming, I'll tell you what I tell my clients: "You CAN do it!"

Now is a great time to start! Supermarkets are overflowing with "mainstream" veggie products that taste great. Armed with some knowledge and an open mind, you can and will feel very satisfied with your new eating style. Try it and sample a refreshing change of taste!

Why Vegetarian?

Vegetarian eating styles have enjoyed increasing popularity, as many recognize the health benefits. Approximately 2.5 percent of the adult population in the United States consistently follows a vegetarian diet. Epidemiological data, as well as large studies, have found that vegetarians have far lower rates of death from heart disease (34 percent lower in vegetarian men, 20 percent lower in vegetarian women). This can be explained in part by vegetarians' lower cholesterol levels and higher intakes of antioxidant vitamins and phytochemicals. Vegetarians also have lower systolic and diastolic blood pressures, with lower rates of hypertension (high blood pressure). Their risk of diabetes and rates of cancer, particularly prostate and colorectal cancers, are also lower. Additionally, vegetarians are less likely to develop dementia, diverticular disease or gallstones. Compared to their meat-eating counterparts, vegetarians also enjoy healthier weights. Studies have consistently found that body mass index (BMI) is lower among vegetarians. This has been explained by differences in nutrient intake (lower fat, saturated fat and protein intake), higher fiber consumption with a higher intake of vegetables, and lower alcohol intake.

While health has been shown to be the most important motivation in choosing a vegetarian eating style, it is not the only one. A 1997 survey showed that religious, spiritual and metaphysical beliefs exert an important influence. "Metaphysical" was defined as "achieving a more proper spiritual or interior balance, often conducive to meditation or higher ideas." The vegetarians questioned claimed that their diets help them to be calmer, more spiritual and clearer in thought. Ethical attitudes play a major role for some, with concerns about animal suffering a major determinant in their food choices. Still others cite efficient use of the world's grain reserves, a theme popularized by Frances Moore Lappé's 1971 book *Diet for a Small Planet.*

There are various types of vegetarians, depending on the extent to which they exclude animal products from their diet. A "vegan," or strict vegetarian, avoids all foods of animal origin. A lacto-ovo vegetarian eats both dairy products and eggs. Some call themselves vegetarians but in fact eat fish and poultry.

Vegetarian diets have been shown to be healthier than the traditional American diet. They are higher in fiber, fruits and vegetables and lower in saturated fat and cholesterol than the nonvegetarian diet. Although vegetarians do not have a greater risk of iron deficiency than nonvegetarians, their diets tend to be lower in iron. The high ascorbic acid content of the diet aids in the absorption of nonheme (vegetable-based) iron present in fruits, vegetables and cereals. Calcium and vitamin D deficiencies are concerns only in vegan diets, in which dairy products are not consumed. In those cases, a source of these nutrients has to be assured.

Vegetarian diets meet and exceed the RDA for protein, although they provide less protein than a diet that includes a meat.

As vitamin B_{12} is found only in foods of animal origin, it may be low in the strict vegetarian or vegan. Reliable sources of vitamin B_{12} include fortified breakfast cereals, soy beverages or vitamin supplements containing B_{12}. So take heart and give it a try. You'll find that a well-planned vegetarian eating style is not only safe and nutritious but highly beneficial from a health perspective!

Making Changes

No one ever said that making changes is easy. In fact, Margaret Mead is quoted as saying, "I'd rather change a man's religion than change his eating habits." The fact that you have purchased this book and are reading this chapter is evidence of your strong intention to improve your health and well-being through yoga and a healthier eating style. Once you understand the goals of the Yoga-Friendly Foods Plan, you have two choices. One is to make BIG changes and do it ALL NOW! Some researchers have found that those willing to make big changes—involving stricter guidelines—achieve a higher degree of success than those who set themselves lesser goals.

The Yoga-Friendly Foods Plan involves eliminating animal flesh (a big step for most people!), eating ten fruits and vegetables a day (most of us can't even manage five a day!) and counting grams of saturated fat to equal 7 percent of your total intake of calories (that means reading labels!).

Undertaking all these BIG changes will help you feel much better NOW—and encourage you to continue! Small, gradual changes in your eating may not help you feel noticeably different as quickly. However, personal styles differ. Most educators believe that adopting SMALL, GRADUAL changes over time leads to further successful goal-setting. They suggest you set yourself one small goal. Pick one that is positive ("I will eat three pieces of fresh fruit today") rather than negative ("I will not eat candy") and measurable. Also pick one that you will be successful doing. Educators would be happy if you decided to eat plant-based meals *every other* day. Better this than to try ALL NOW and fail miserably. Do what feels right for you . . . tiptoe or jump in . . . small and gradual or ALL NOW!

Other suggestions for improving your chances of success include monitoring your progress. You might want to keep a food diary and record your daily intake, including targeted nutrients like grams of saturated fat. Get the support of friends and/or family, believe in your ability to eat healthier, have patience, be adventurous and try new foods and recipes, bearing in mind that you may not like everything but that it's worth finding out. Do the best you can. Practice positive self-talk, learn from your mistakes, take your time and plan ahead.

Set the stage for success by surrounding yourself with healthful foods and avoid deprivation. Know that there will be bumps in the road ahead but KEEP TRYING! One does not *arrive* at a healthy eating style or a healthy weight and then go back to old, bad habits. This is a lifelong journey of many choices. You are lucky to be taking this opportunity now to create a healthier eating style and a healthier you!

Weight Management

$\mathcal{L}$ook around! It's obvious that Americans are getting bigger, with one in three adults classified as obese and nearly two-thirds either overweight or obese. Our kids are in trouble, too, with one in five now overweight.

Are you overweight or obese? One measure, which eliminates reliance on frame size, is called the body mass index, or BMI. Check the chart on page 220 to determine your BMI. Locate your height in inches on the vertical axis and move across to find your weight in pounds. Move to the top for your BMI. A BMI of 19–24.9 is associated with the lowest health risk. A BMI of 25–29.9 is considered overweight, and over 30 is classified as obese.

Body-fat distribution is also important, especially in predicting your risk of cardiovascular disease. To determine if you are an apple (higher risk) or a pear (lower risk), measure your waist at its smallest part. Women who measure greater than 35 inches and men greater than 40 inches are considered to be at increased cardiovascular risk (apple shape).

If your weight and/or weight distribution is worrisome and you are *ready* to make changes, setting a reasonable weight goal is an important first step. *Small changes* in weight can make a big difference in health. Studies show that a 10 percent decrease in weight can be sufficient to lower blood sugar, blood pressure and cholesterol. So set your goal for a "healthier weight target," or 10 percent less than you weigh now. This means that if you are a woman 5'4" tall and 170 pounds, your healthier weight target is 153 pounds, despite the fact that weight charts may show your ideal weight as 120 to 135 pounds. Slow and steady wins the race. Why rush? A weight loss rate of 1 to 4 pounds a month for women and 2 to 8 pounds a month for men is reasonable. If you have been steadily putting on weight over the past few years, maintaining a stable weight for a few months may be a more realistic goal for you.

After considering your healthier weight target, make an effort to banish the word *diet* from your thoughts! "Diet" implies denial and restriction. It is something that you aren't expected to stay on . . . you're off and then you're on again. It's a vicious cycle.

You've chosen the Yoga-Friendly Foods Plan as a healthier eating style. I like to think of it as "gentle nutrition." There are many wonderful and tasty foods to choose from. It should not be too restrictive. First, embrace the abundance of fruits and vegetables. Fill up and don't go hungry. Take care of yourself by making soups and salads and cutting up fresh fruit. Plan ahead and surround yourself with lots of healthy foods. Experiment with protein-rich foods: soy-based meat alternatives, beans and tofu. Try new whole grains. Balance your day with a sprinkling of unsaturated fats and sweets or alcohol, if desired. Read labels and key in on important items such as saturated fat. With regular exercise and healthy eating, slow, gradual weight loss will just happen!

Help! I Need Limits!

There are those of us who may not be able to lose weight without guidance. It is simply a matter of taking in fewer calories than you burn in a day. Work on the "output" side carefully. People who have successfully lost weight and kept it off for a number of years cite one key factor: They exercise almost daily (to the equivalent

FIND YOUR OWN BODY MASS INDEX

Body Mass Index	19	20	21	22	23	24	25	26	27	28	29	30	31	32	33	34	35
Height (inches)	Body Weight (pounds)																
58	91	96	100	105	110	115	119	124	129	134	138	143	148	153	158	162	167
59	94	99	104	109	114	119	124	128	133	138	143	148	153	158	163	168	173
60	97	102	107	112	118	123	128	133	138	143	148	153	158	163	168	174	179
61	100	106	111	116	122	127	132	137	143	148	153	158	164	169	174	180	185
62	104	109	115	120	126	131	136	142	147	153	158	164	169	175	180	186	191
63	107	113	118	124	130	135	141	146	152	158	163	169	175	180	186	191	197
64	110	116	122	128	134	140	145	151	157	163	169	174	180	186	192	197	204
65	114	120	126	132	138	144	150	156	162	168	174	180	186	192	198	204	210
66	118	124	130	136	142	148	155	161	167	173	179	186	192	198	204	210	216
67	121	127	134	140	146	153	159	166	172	178	185	191	198	204	211	217	223
68	125	131	138	144	151	158	164	171	177	184	190	197	203	210	216	223	230
69	128	135	142	149	155	162	169	176	182	189	196	203	209	216	223	230	236
70	132	139	146	153	160	167	174	181	188	195	202	209	216	222	229	236	243
71	136	143	150	157	165	172	179	186	193	200	208	215	222	229	236	243	250
72	140	147	154	162	169	177	184	191	199	206	213	221	228	235	242	250	258
73	144	151	159	166	174	182	189	197	204	212	219	227	235	242	250	257	265
74	148	155	163	171	179	186	194	202	210	218	225	233	241	249	256	264	272
75	152	160	168	176	184	192	200	208	216	224	232	240	248	256	264	272	279
76	156	164	172	180	189	197	205	213	221	230	238	246	254	263	271	279	287

Locate your height in inches, move across to find your weight, then up to your Body Mass Index.

of walking twenty miles per week). Find a physical activity that you enjoy and get moving!

Next, take a look at the portion of each yoga-friendly food recommended for certain calorie levels. Refer to the chart on page 222. Most women lose weight on 1,200–1,500 calories a day, while men lose weight on 1,500–1,800 calories. Often, it is a matter of redefining your idea of a "serving." For example, a serving of starch is equal to one slice of bread (a bagel store bagel is about four to five servings) or a half cup of pasta (a restaurant portion is about six servings). Take out that measuring cup and fill any empty spaces on your plate with more veggies! I keep a large plate on my desk at work to show clients that vegetables should fill half the plate, with one-quarter taken up by protein-rich foods and the remaining quarter by a whole grain.

How Much Is One Portion or Serving?

FRUIT (60 CALORIES EACH)

- 1 piece, or a handful of fresh fruit
- 1 cup chopped
- ½ cup canned (no sugar added)
- 2 Tbsp raisins
- half a 9-inch banana
- 3 prunes
- ½ cup juice

VEGETABLES (25 CALORIES EACH)

- ½ cup cooked
- 1 cup raw
- 1 cup juice

WHOLE GRAINS (80 CALORIES EACH)

- 1 slice bread
- ½ cup pasta, rice, corn, or peas

HELP! I NEED LIMITS!	HOW MUCH CAN I EAT?				
	Calories				
SERVINGS OF:	1,200	1,500	1,800	2,100	2,500
Fruit	4	5	5	5	5
Vegetables	6	5	5	5	5
Protein Rich	2	2	3	3	4
Dairy/Soy Alt	2	2	3	3	3
Fat 20%	1 fat serving	1 fat serving	2 fat servings	2 fat servings	3 fat servings
Whole Grain	3 whole grain	5 whole grain	5 whole grain	7 whole grain	10 whole grain
OR:					
Fat 30%	2 fat servings	2 fat servings	3 fat servings	4 fat servings	5 fat servings
Whole Grain	2 whole grain	4 whole grain	4 whole grain	5 whole grain	6 whole grain
Saturated Fat	9g	12g	14g	16g	19g
Fiber	25g+	25g+	25g+	25g+	25g+
Extras (Sweets or Alcohol)	100 calories	100 calories	150 calories	150 calories	200 calories

- ¾ oz cereal
- ¾ oz crackers
- 6-inch corn tortilla
- half a 6-inch whole wheat pita
- 1 3-oz potato
- 1 cup winter squash

PROTEIN-RICH FOODS (100 CALORIES EACH)
- 1 veggie burger, veggie hot dog or veggie sausage patty
- 1 cup beans
- 4 oz tofu
- 4 egg whites
- 1 cup egg substitute
- 1 whole egg (1–2 per week limit)
- ¾ cup non-fat cottage cheese
- ½ cup non-fat ricotta
- ½–¾ cup "burger" meat
- 5 slices soy luncheon meat
- other meat alternatives in a portion to equal 100 calories

DAIRY AND SOY ALTERNATIVES (80 CALORIES)
- 1 cup non-fat or 1% milk
- 1 cup soy milk
- 1 cup non-fat yogurt
- 2 oz non-fat cheese or soy cheese (reduced or low-fat cheeses occasionally, to stay within saturated-fat goal)

FATS AND OILS (135 CALORIES)
- 1 Tbsp olive or canola oil (preferred for home use)
- 1 Tbsp peanut or sesame oil
- 2 Tbsp natural peanut butter
- 1 oz or ⅓ cup nuts
- ¼ avocado

- 2 Tbsp seeds or tahini
- 2 Tbsp salad dressing
- 1–2 Tbsp trans fat–free margarine (if light, check the portion to equal 15 grams fat)
- 1 Tbsp mayonnaise or 3 Tbsp light mayonnaise
- olives, any kind, amount to equal 15 grams of fat

ALCOHOL
- 5 oz wine
- 12 oz beer
- 1½ oz hard liquor (1 for women, 2 for men daily)

SWEETS
- Fat-free sweets in a portion equal to 100–200 calories, depending on calorie target (if not fat-free, count the saturated fat in your daily allowance)

READING FOOD LABELS

Need a nutrition degree to help you decipher food labels? The process can be less daunting if you take it one step at a time!

Before we begin, keep in mind your daily limits of some important nutrients. As total fat and saturated fat are based on calorie goals, locate your needs in the chart below. While we are not "counting" calories, most women need 1,200–1,500 for weight loss (depending on your age and activity level) and 1,800–2,000 a day for weight maintenance. Men need about 1,500–1,800 calories for weight loss and 2,000–2,500 for weight maintenance. Find the appropriate calorie level and determine your total fat and saturated fat limits.

Calories	1,200	1,500	1,800	2,000	2,500
Total fat (g) 20%–30%	27–40	33–50	40–60	44–67	55–83
Sat fat (g) 7%	9	12	14	16	19
Sodium (mg)	3,000*	3,000	3,000	3,000	3,000
Fiber (g)	25+**	25+	25+	25+	25+

*Sodium guidelines of 2,400 mg per day are recommended by the American Heart Association. The "DASH" trial used 3,000 mg per day for effective blood pressure lowering. If you do not have high blood pressure, advanced or congestive heart failure, kidney or liver disease, a strict limitation of sodium may not be necessary. Check with your physician for your individual sodium goal.

**Fiber recommendations of more than 25 grams per day are proposed by the American Institute for Cancer Research. Levels as high as 50 grams per day have been used successfully to lower blood glucose levels. How much you are able to tolerate depends on your current intake and the sensitivity of your stomach. When increasing fiber intake, drink plenty of fluids.

Looking at Labels

As you look at labels and try to determine whether to purchase a particular food, it is important to remember that all foods can fit into your individualized plan. It depends on your health history, other foods consumed that day or week, portion size and your nutrition goals. A generally "off-limits" candy bar with 5 grams of saturated fat can fit into most meal plans *occasionally*. Try to work your favorite foods in rather than "cheat."

Step One

Note the *serving size* (not usually the whole can/package!). Just once, take out measuring utensils and see what a half cup of pasta, 1 cup of cereal or 2 tablespoons of salad dressing looks like. The serving size noted on the label may be different from the portions you are used to eating.

Step Two

Note the *total fat,* in grams, for the serving listed. Consider this in relation to your daily limits. Fat is calorically dense, at 9 calories per gram, compared to carbohydrates (4 calories per gram) and protein (4 calories per gram). Some studies have found that people have better success at managing their weight by curbing their fat levels. Exceeding your daily fat allowance may impact your weight but not your blood cholesterol level, *if* the fat is saturated (see below).

Step Three

Note the *saturated fat,* in grams, for the serving listed. Saturated fat increases the "bad" LDL cholesterol in your blood. Do not exceed your daily limits, especially if you have heart disease. A small vegetable pot pie that contains 16 grams of saturated fat will not easily fit into most healthful eating styles. Compare labels for a better choice.

Step Four

Trans fatty acids are another kind of bad fat lurking in foods. These fats act just like saturated fat, raising the level of LDL cholesterol. Unfortunately, the FDA does not require labels to inform us of the amount of trans fat contained in a product. However, reading through the ingredients list will help you identify trans fats. They are listed as *hydrogenated oil, partially hydrogenated oil, margarine* or *shortening*.

While it is best to avoid products containing trans fatty acids, favorite foods containing small amounts may be enjoyed occasionally. Count all the fat contained in the serving as saturated fat, to assume the worst. For instance, if a favorite cracker contains 3 grams total fat and 1 gram saturated fat per a ten-cracker serving, count the ten crackers as having 3 grams of saturated fat.

Step Five

Note the milligrams of *sodium* and the grams of *fiber* per serving. Compare products and select the lower-sodium and higher-fiber options.

❀ CHOLESTEROL ❀

You don't need to be overly concerned about *cholesterol,* as the plant-based, Yoga-friendly eating plan is naturally low in cholesterol (cholesterol is found only in foods of animal origin). Egg yolks are limited to one or two per week to prevent heart disease, or are not allowed if you have heart disease. There is a small amount of cholesterol in dairy products, but in the amounts recommended your cholesterol intake will be low. Additionally, don't be confused by the percentages listed on the label. These percentages are more liberal guidelines based on a 2,000-calorie and a 2,500-calorie eating plan. Although your label-reading efforts may take some time in the beginning, shopping will go faster as you become familiar with them. A thorough reading will only be necessary when deciding whether or not to purchase a new product you haven't tried before.

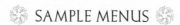 SAMPLE MENUS

Sunday

Breakfast	Lunch	Dinner	Snack
Chopped vegetable frittata with soy sausage Whole wheat toast with jam Fresh orange slice Non-fat milk	Veggie burger with soy cheese on whole wheat bun Lettuce and tomato Vegetarian baked beans Fresh apple	Gingery Chinese vegetables with sautéed tofu Brown rice Fresh pineapple chunks	Sorbet with fresh raspberries

Monday

Breakfast	Lunch	Dinner	Snack
High fiber cereal with banana Chopped walnuts Non-fat milk	Soy luncheon meat sandwich on whole wheat bread Crunchy carrot and jicama strips Fresh strawberries	Pasta fagioli Baby greens with vinaigrette Jell-O with mandarin oranges	Non-fat light yogurt

Tuesday

Breakfast	Lunch	Dinner	Snack
Oatmeal with raisins Non-fat milk	Japanese tofu bowl (broccoli, cabbage, tofu and rice) Green grapes	Whole wheat couscous pilaf with garbanzo beans Spinach salad with light ranch dressing Fresh sliced mango	Cantaloupe wedges Non-fat yogurt

Wednesday

Breakfast	Lunch	Dinner	Snack
Whole wheat toast with natural peanut butter Banana Non-fat milk	Pea soup with carrots, celery and potatoes Natural rye cracker with soy cheese Fresh cherries	Winter vegetable chili Homemade cornbread Fresh pear	Sliced fresh kiwi

Thursday

Breakfast	Lunch	Dinner	Snack
French toast (made with egg substitute) with syrup Grapefruit sections Non-fat milk	Hummus in a whole wheat pita Cucumber salad Cherry tomatoes Fresh nectarine	Taco salad made with veggie ground beef and soy cheese Black beans Roasted corn Avocado slices Fresh pineapple	Cinnamon applesauce and a fig bar

Friday

Breakfast	Lunch	Dinner	Snack
Non-fat cottage cheese/fresh fruit plate Whole wheat English muffin with jelly Non-fat milk	Vegetable salad with garbanzo beans with oil and vinegar Non-fat croutons Fresh orange	Eggplant Parmesan with zucchini, mushrooms, and carrots Whole wheat roll Fresh grapes	Dried apricots and almonds

Saturday

Breakfast	Lunch	Dinner	Snack
One half whole-wheat bagel with lite veggie cream cheese Blueberries Non-fat milk	Minestrone soup with wheat crackers Veggie hot dog Strawberries	Barbecued vegetables with brown rice Spinach salad with mandarin oranges and peanuts Homemade carrot cake	Non-fat plain yogurt with no-sugar-added canned peaches

Sunday

Breakfast	Lunch	Dinner	Snack
Sautéed egg white omelet with spinach and mushrooms Natural applesauce Fresh raspberries Non-fat milk	Bean and soy cheese burrito Non-fat sour cream Mixed green salad with non-fat dressing Tomato wedges Mixed fruit cup	Broccoli-stuffed shells Steamed asparagus Watermelon cubes	Hot cocoa with non-fat milk Marshmallows

Monday

Breakfast	Lunch	Dinner	Snack
Hot steel-cut oatmeal Walnuts Whole grapefruit Non-fat milk	Soy grilled cheese with trans fat–free margarine Cucumber, onion, and green bean salad Fresh apple	Cajun red beans and rice Corn on the cob Angel cake Fresh strawberries	Frozen grapes

Tuesday

Breakfast	Lunch	Dinner	Snack
Non-fat plain yogurt with berries Whole wheat toast with avocado Non-fat milk	Natural peanut butter with jam on whole wheat bread Cherry tomatoes Baked potato chips Fresh banana	Baked potato with steamed broccoli, soy cheese, and veggie chili Baby greens salad with non-fat dressing Cantaloupe half	Non-fat pudding cup

Wednesday

Breakfast	Lunch	Dinner	Snack
Scrambled egg substitute with veggie Canadian bacon Whole wheat waffle with syrup Fresh blueberries Non-fat milk	Homemade vegetable soup Whole wheat crackers Fresh apple	Grilled portobello mushroom Vegetable skewer Wild rice Natural canned fruit cocktail	Everyday banana bread

Thursday

Breakfast	Lunch	Dinner	Snack
High-fiber cereal with chopped walnuts Fresh banana Non-fat milk	Black beans and rice Chopped fresh tomatoes Low-fat cole slaw Fresh pineapple chunks	Spaghetti with tomato sauce Veggie meatballs Sautéed zucchini and summer squash Fresh peach	Non-fat yogurt

Friday

Breakfast	Lunch	Dinner	Snack
Whole wheat toast with soy cheese Grapefruit sections Non-fat milk	Lentil soup Fresh red and yellow pepper strips Whole wheat crackers Sliced mango	Vegetarian tamale pie Fresh apple	Apricots Low-fat graham crackers

Saturday

Breakfast	Lunch	Dinner	Snack
Bread pudding made with egg substitute Raisins Honeydew melon wedge Non-fat milk	Ratatouille Romaine salad with non-fat Caesar dressing Fresh plums	Spinach-cheese bake Steamed vegetable medley Whole wheat roll Fresh pear	Non-fat ice cream Chocolate syrup

Favorite Everyday Recipes

Appetizers

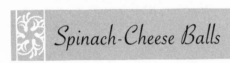

Spinach-Cheese Balls

A great appetizer for company. Prepare a day ahead and bake fresh for the occasion.

MAKES 20–25 ONE-INCH BALLS

NUTRITIONAL ANALYSIS: CALORIES 128 FAT 3G SAT FAT 1.5G CHOLESTEROL 3MG
PROTEIN 10G CARBOHYDRATE 16G FIBER 3G SODIUM 312MG

> *10-oz package chopped spinach, frozen (thawed and drained)*
> *½ cup egg substitute or 3 egg whites*
> *¾ cup bread crumbs*
> *⅓ cup Parmesan cheese, non-fat if desired*
> *¼ cup finely minced onion*
> *½ tsp poultry seasoning*
> *¼ tsp garlic powder*
> *⅛ tsp pepper*

Preheat oven to 350 degrees. Combine and mix all ingredients. Shape into one-inch balls. Place on un-greased cookie sheet and bake for 15–20 minutes. Serve hot with honey mustard or other favorite sauce.

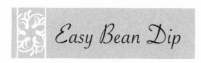

Easy Bean Dip

*K*eep some cans of non-fat refried beans on hand and you are ready for a party!

SERVES 6

NUTRITIONAL ANALYSIS: (SERVING SIZE ⅓ CUP) CALORIES 60 FAT 0G SAT FAT 0MG
CHOLESTEROL 0MG PROTEIN 4G CARBOHYDRATE 11G FIBER 3G SODIUM 275MG

16-oz can non-fat refried beans
1 Tbsp cumin
2 Tbsp salsa
1 green onion, minced

Mix all ingredients in a microwave-safe serving bowl. Microwave on High 4–5 minutes. Serve with baked corn chips.

Garbanzo Bean Spread

A non-fat version of hummus, this Middle Eastern spread is made with non-fat yogurt rather than high-fat tahini and olive oil. Serve on whole grain pita with cucumbers or enjoy as a dip for fresh vegetables.

SERVES 6

NUTRITIONAL ANALYSIS: (SERVING SIZE ¼ CUP) CALORIES 50 FAT 1G SAT FAT 0G
CHOLESTEROL 0MG PROTEIN 6G CARBOHYDRATE 11G FIBER 4G SODIUM 74MG

16-oz can lower-sodium garbanzo beans (rinsed and drained)
2 Tbsp water

½ tsp garlic powder

1 Tbsp minced fresh parsley

juice of 1 fresh lemon

paprika to taste

Put all ingredients, except paprika, in food processor and process until smooth. Sprinkle with paprika and serve.

 ## Elegant Artichoke Pockets

𝒯hese appetizers only look like you worked hard. Great for company!

SERVES 8

NUTRITIONAL ANALYSIS: (SERVING SIZE 3 WRAPPERS) CALORIES 134 FAT 6G SAT FAT 1G CHOLESTEROL 7MG PROTEIN 4G CARBOHYDRATE 16G FIBER 3.5G SODIUM 385MG

---

2 13-oz cans artichoke hearts (rinsed and drained)

⅓ cup light mayonnaise

¼ cup freshly grated Parmesan cheese

1 red pepper, minced

5 Tbsp (half a 4-oz can) chopped ripe olives

½ tsp garlic powder

24 wonton wrappers

Blend artichoke hearts, mayo and Parmesan cheese in food processor until smooth. Mix in red pepper, olives and garlic powder. Divide evenly between wrappers. Pull wrappers up at corners and press to close and create a pocket. Bake at 350 degrees for 15 minutes. Serve warm.

Soups and Salads

Black Bean Salad

*T*his salad is easy to toss together with ingredients you may already have in your kitchen.

SERVES 4

NUTRITIONAL ANALYSIS: (SERVING SIZE ¾ CUP) CALORIES 135 FAT 0G SAT FAT 0G
CHOLESTEROL 0MG PROTEIN 8G CARBOHYDRATE 26G FIBER 9G SODIUM 191MG

---

1 16-oz can lower-sodium black beans, rinsed and drained

1 cup chopped fresh Roma tomatoes

½ cup frozen corn, thawed

½ cup chopped green pepper

2 Tbsp minced red onion

¼ cup salsa

juice of 1 lime

Mix all ingredients. Chill and serve as a side dish.

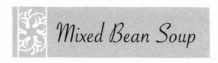

Mixed Bean Soup

A thick, hearty soup . . . delicious as a meal. Serve with a salad and crusty bread.

SERVES 8

NUTRITIONAL ANALYSIS: (SERVING SIZE ⅛ RECIPE) CALORIES 302 FAT 2G SAT FAT 0G
CHOLESTEROL 0MG PROTEIN 17G CARBOHYDRATE 58G FIBER 12G SODIUM 281MG

---

20 oz (about 2 cups) assorted dried beans

6 cups or more chicken broth, stock or water

28-oz can chopped tomatoes

1 medium onion, minced

3 stalks celery, chopped

2 carrots, chopped

2 bay leaves

½ tsp marjoram

½ tsp basil

½ tsp coriander

¼ tsp savory

¼ tsp thyme

1½ tsp chopped garlic

¼ cup chopped fresh parsley

fresh ground pepper

Rinse and sort the beans. Place in large pot with enough cold water to cover generously. Let stand overnight. Drain beans and return to pot. Add 6 cups liquid and bring to a boil. Reduce heat and simmer, covered, for 1 hour. Add tomatoes, onion, celery, carrots, spices and garlic to soup and simmer, uncovered, for about 1 hour. If necessary, add more liquid. Add parsley and pepper and serve.

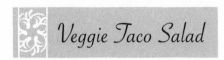

Veggie Taco Salad

A taco salad made with "veggie" ground beef . . . you won't even miss the meat!

MAKES 2 LARGE SERVINGS

NUTRITIONAL ANALYSIS: (Serving size ½ recipe) Calories 408 Fat 3.5g Sat Fat 0g
Cholesterol 0mg Protein 30g Carbohydrate 71g Fiber 23g Sodium 748mg

---

> *1 cup (half 12-oz package) veggie ground round, taco flavor*
> *4 cups mixed greens*
> *8–10 cherry tomatoes, halved*
> *¼ red onion, minced*
> *½ green pepper, chopped*
> *1 yellow or red pepper, chopped*
> *½ cup frozen corn, thawed*
> *1 16-oz can lower-sodium black beans, rinsed and drained*
> *4 Tbsp sliced black olives*
> *¼ cup salsa*
> *1 serving baked corn chips (1 oz or about 18 chips)*

Sauté veggie ground round for 5–10 minutes to heat thoroughly. Place other in-gredients except salsa and chips in large serving bowl. Top with warmed ground round, salsa and "crunched" corn chips. Divide and conquer!

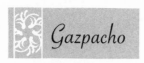

Gazpacho

This is an enjoyable way to eat your veggies!

SERIES 4

NUTRITIONAL ANALYSIS: CALORIES 56 FAT 0G SAT FAT 0G CHOLESTEROL 0MG
PROTEIN 2G CARBOHYDRATE 11G FIBER 2G SODIUM 258MG

---

1 cup tomato juice

1 cup low-sodium tomato juice

3 tomatoes, chopped

1 green pepper, minced

1 cucumber, peeled, seeded and chopped

½ onion, minced

juice of ½ lemon and 1 lime

1 Tbsp wine vinegar

½ tsp each tarragon and basil

¼ cup minced fresh parsley

dash Tabasco

dash ground cumin

black pepper to taste

Combine all ingredients and chill at least 2 hours. Garnish with yogurt or non-fat sour cream and serve.

Vegetarian Tamale Pie

A tasty and filling meal that is easy to throw together.

SERVES 4

NUTRITIONAL ANALYSIS: (SERVING SIZE ¼ RECIPE) CALORIES 311 FAT 2G SAT FAT 0G
CHOLESTEROL 0MG PROTEIN 13G CARBOHYDRATE 65G FIBER 12G SODIUM 734MG

PIE
½ cup chopped onion
½ cup chopped green pepper
17-oz can no-salt-added corn
16-oz can pinto beans, rinsed
4-oz can green chilies
6-oz can tomato sauce
¼ cup salsa
½ tsp cumin
2 Tbsp chili powder

TOPPING
1¼ cups water
½ cup cornmeal
⅛ tsp salt (optional)

Preheat oven to 375 degrees. Sprinkle onion, green pepper, corn, beans and green chilies into an 8x8-inch baking dish sprayed with nonstick cooking spray. Stir in tomato sauce, salsa, cumin and chili powder.

In a small saucepan combine water, cornmeal and salt, if desired. Bring to a boil, then reduce heat and stir for about 1 minute, until it thickens slightly. Spoon over bean/vegetable mixture for topping. Bake for 40–50 minutes.

Note: For variation, add 2½-oz can sliced black olives.

 ## Sautéed Tofu with Gingery Chinese Vegetables

*E*njoy the freshness of these crisp Chinese veggies. It's quick and easy . . . after the chopping is done!

SERVES 4

NUTRITIONAL ANALYSIS: (SERVING SIZE 3 OZ TOFU AND 2 CUPS VEGGIES)
CALORIES 215 FAT 12G SAT FAT 1.3G CHOLESTEROL 0MG PROTEIN 12G
CARBOHYDRATE 16G FIBER 5G SODIUM 162MG

½ cup minced onion

2–3 cloves garlic, minced

3–4 Tbsp shredded fresh ginger

2–3 Tbsp sesame oil

1 cup sliced mushrooms

1 cup shredded carrot

1 cup mung bean sprouts

1 cup sliced celery

3 cups chopped bok choy

1 cup Chinese pea pods

2 cups broccoli florets

⅓ cup peanuts, if desired

soy sauce to taste

12 oz firm tofu, cut into bite-size pieces

In a large sauté pan or wok, sauté onion, garlic and ginger in sesame oil for 5 minutes. Add mushrooms and carrots and continue sautéing for 5 more minutes. Add remaining ingredients, except tofu, and continue cooking 5–10 more minutes until veggies are crisp-tender. Add tofu to heat quickly and serve. Enjoy with rice.

Barbequed Vegetables

*M*ake vegetables taste special!

SERVES 2

NUTRITIONAL ANALYSIS: (SERVING SIZE ½ RECIPE) CALORIES 230 FAT 0G
SAT FAT 0G CHOLESTEROL 0MG PROTEIN 7G CARBOHYDRATE 49G FIBER 8G
SODIUM 425MG (DEPENDING ON SAUCE)

---

4 new potatoes, cut into bite-size pieces

1 onion, sliced

1 zucchini, sliced

1 summer squash, sliced

1 green pepper, sliced

1 red pepper, sliced

8 or more large mushrooms

½ cup BBQ sauce

Preheat oven to 425 degrees. Spray a 9x13-inch baking pan with nonstick cooking spray. Precook potatoes slightly by microwaving them for 3 minutes on High. Put all veggies into the prepared pan and brush with BBQ sauce. Bake for 15 minutes and finish off under the broiler for 5 minutes to blacken slightly. Serve with basmati rice and a salad.

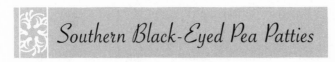

Southern Black-Eyed Pea Patties

*A*n interesting twist to traditional veggie burgers. Serve in a whole wheat pita pocket with tomato, cucumber and non-fat sour cream.

SERVES 6

NUTRITIONAL ANALYSIS: (SERVING SIZE 1 PATTY) CALORIES 158 FAT 3G SAT FAT 0G
CHOLESTEROL 0MG PROTEIN 8.5G CARBOHYDRATE 20G FIBER 2.5G SODIUM 126MG

⅔ *cup oats*

2½ cups black-eyed peas, cooked

3 green onions, sliced

2 egg whites

1 tsp cumin

1½ tsp chili powder

⅛ tsp cayenne pepper

¼ tsp salt

1 Tbsp canola oil

Process oats in food processor to a powder. Take out and reserve 3 Tbsp. Add all ingredients except oil to the processor and process to a thick paste. Make 6 patties. Roll in reserved oat powder and sauté in canola oil in a nonstick skillet. Cook through and brown on each side.

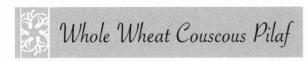

Whole Wheat Couscous Pilaf

*C*ouscous is a grain made of semolina or other ground cracked wheat. It originated in North Africa and is very popular in France, where it is used like rice. In this dish, couscous is mixed with chopped vegetables and garbanzo beans to serve as a main dish.

SERVES 2

NUTRITIONAL ANALYSIS: (SERVING SIZE ½ RECIPE) CALORIES 553 FAT 10G SAT FAT 1G
CHOLESTEROL 0MG PROTEIN 23G CARBOHYDRATE 94G FIBER 13G SODIUM 330MG

1 cup fat-free vegetable broth

¾ cup whole wheat couscous

1 Tbsp canola or olive oil

1 clove garlic, minced

1 cup or more broccoli florets

1–2 carrots, shredded

8 mushrooms or more, sliced

2 green onions, sliced

½ cup frozen peas

1 cup lower-sodium garbanzo beans, rinsed

Bring broth to a boil. Add couscous. Remove from heat and let stand for 5 minutes, covered. In a sauté pan, add the oil, then sauté garlic and add vegetables and beans. Stir-fry for 5–8 minutes. Combine veggie mixture and couscous and serve.

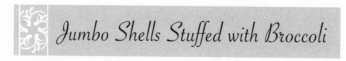

Jumbo Shells Stuffed with Broccoli

*G*ood enough to serve company!

SERVES 6

NUTRITIONAL ANALYSIS: (SERVING SIZE 5 SHELLS) CALORIES 223 FAT 2.3G SAT FAT 1G CHOLESTEROL 5MG PROTEIN 20G CARBOHYDRATE 36G FIBER 4G SODIUM 198MG (DEPENDING ON SAUCE)

---

1 package large pasta shells

15 oz non-fat ricotta cheese

4 Tbsp freshly grated Parmesan cheese

2 egg whites

¼ tsp garlic powder

½ tsp nutmeg

¼ tsp black pepper

½ tsp oregano

2½ cups broccoli florets, steamed and minced (or 10-oz frozen package)

4 cups tomato sauce (use low-sodium, if desired)

1 cup or more sliced fresh mushrooms

Preheat oven to 350 degrees. Cook shells according to package directions. In a large bowl, mix cheeses, egg whites and spices. Stir in broccoli. Use tablespoon to fill shells.

In a 9x13-inch glass baking pan prepared with nonstick cooking spray, coat with one-third of the tomato sauce. Arrange shells in the pan and pour in the rest of the sauce and the mushrooms. Bake for 35–40 minutes.

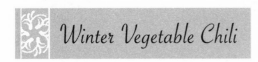 *Winter Vegetable Chili*

$\mathcal{A}$ warm and filling dish.

SERVES 6

NUTRITIONAL ANALYSIS: (SERVING SIZE ⅙ RECIPE) CALORIES 418 FAT 4G SAT FAT 500MG CHOLESTEROL 0MG PROTEIN 20G CARBOHYDRATE 81G FIBER 17G SODIUM 443MG

1 onion, chopped

1 green pepper, chopped

2 cloves garlic, minced

1 Tbsp oil

4 small new potatoes, cut into bite-size pieces

1 butternut squash, peeled and chopped

2 carrots, sliced thin

2 16-oz cans no-salt-added chopped tomatoes

6-oz can tomato paste

4-oz can diced green chilies

29-oz can pinto beans, rinsed

16-oz can small white beans, rinsed

1 cup frozen corn

1 tsp oregano

2–4 Tbsp chili powder

water

In a large sauté pan, sauté onion, green pepper and garlic in oil. Add rest of ingredients and cook over medium heat, adding water as needed, for 45 minutes or until veggies are done.

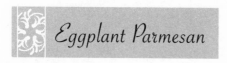

Eggplant Parmesan

*A*uthentic taste without gobs of grease. The big difference is that the eggplant is breaded then *baked*, not fried!

SERVES 6

NUTRITIONAL ANALYSIS: (SERVING SIZE ⅙ OF RECIPE) CALORIES 222 FAT 5.5G SAT FAT 2G CHOLESTEROL 10MG PROTEIN 14G CARBOHYDRATE 28G FIBER 6G SODIUM 627MG

2 egg whites

1 large eggplant, peeled and sliced

1 cup bread crumbs

26-oz jar tomato sauce

2 carrots, shredded

1 zucchini, chopped

1 summer squash, chopped

½ lb mushrooms, sliced

4 oz low-fat mozzarella cheese, shredded

2 Tbsp freshly grated Parmesan cheese

Preheat oven to 375 degrees. Mix egg whites in a bowl, dip eggplant slices, then cover in bread crumbs. Put in a 9x13-inch glass baking dish prepared with nonstick cooking spray. Bake for 30 minutes. Remove from oven. Pour sauce over eggplant, sprinkle with veggies and resume baking for 20 minutes. Add cheeses and bake for 10 minutes more, until cheese is melted. Total baking time is 1 hour.

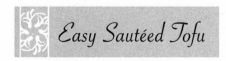 *Easy Sautéed Tofu*

SERVES 3

NUTRITIONAL ANALYSIS: (SERVING SIZE 4 SLICES) CALORIES 140 FAT 10G SAT FAT 1.5G
CHOLESTEROL 0MG PROTEIN 10G CARBOHYDRATE 2G FIBER 1.5G SODIUM 188MG

---

1 lb extra-firm tofu
½ Tbsp canola oil
½ Tbsp sesame oil
Garlic and ginger powder to taste
Low-sodium soy sauce to taste

Drain tofu. Place on cutting board and cut into 12 slices. Wipe both oils on a large sauté pan. Place tofu in pan and sauté about 5 minutes on each side until brown. Dust lightly with garlic and ginger powder and sprinkle with soy sauce during cooking.

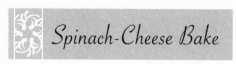

Spinach-Cheese Bake

*E*asy to prepare and always a favorite. Serve as a brunch entrée with salad and whole grain bread.

SERVES 4

NUTRITIONAL ANALYSIS: CALORIES 245 FAT 4.5G SAT FAT 3G CHOLESTEROL 25MG
PROTEIN 37G CARBOHYDRATE 14G FIBER 2.5G SODIUM 790MG

10-oz package frozen chopped spinach, thawed and drained

4 egg whites or 1 cup egg substitute

16 oz non-fat cottage cheese

8 oz shredded low-fat Cheddar cheese or soy cheese

4 Tbsp flour

¼ tsp garlic powder

black pepper to taste

2 Tbsp sliced almonds (optional)

Preheat oven to 350 degrees. Mix all ingredients, except almonds, together and spread in an 8x8-inch baking dish prepared with nonstick spray. Bake for 40–45 minutes (during final 10 minutes, top with almonds) or until knife inserted in center comes out clean. Cool for 10 minutes and serve.

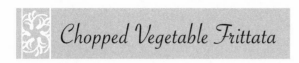

Chopped Vegetable Frittata

*G*reat for a late, lazy breakfast or brunch.

SERVES 2

NUTRITIONAL ANALYSIS: (SERVING SIZE ½ RECIPE) CALORIES 224 FAT 4G SAT FAT 0G
CHOLESTEROL 0MG PROTEIN 18G CARBOHYDRATE 30G FIBER 21G SODIUM 668MG

---

2 green onions, minced

1 tomato, chopped

½ red pepper, chopped

1 green pepper, chopped

1–2 cups sliced mushrooms

1 cup cooked and sliced potato

½ cucumber, peeled and sliced

4-oz can green chilies

8 oz egg substitute

½ tsp garlic powder

¼ tsp white pepper

¼ tsp salt

Prepare a sauté pan with nonstick cooking spray. Sauté all vegetables until crisp-tender. Pour egg substitute over the vegetables, add spices and cook, covered, over low to medium heat until egg is fully cooked and fluffy.

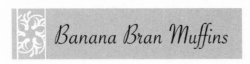

Banana Bran Muffins

This recipe uses those "spotted" bananas! Enjoy for breakfast or anytime!

MAKES 12 MUFFINS

NUTRITIONAL ANALYSIS: (SERVING SIZE 1 MUFFIN) CALORIES 145 FAT 3G SAT FAT 0G
CHOLESTEROL 0MG PROTEIN 3G CARBOHYDRATE 29G FIBER 3G SODIUM 203MG

---

2 ripe bananas

2½ cups bran flakes cereal

1 cup non-fat milk

2 Tbsp canola oil

2 egg whites

1 tsp vanilla extract

1 cup flour

⅓–½ cup sugar

1 Tbsp baking powder

1 tsp cinnamon

¼ cup raisins, if desired

Preheat oven to 375 degrees. In a large mixing bowl, mash bananas with a fork, stir in the remaining ingredients in the order listed and mix well. Prepare a muffin tin with nonstick cooking spray. Divide batter among 12 muffins. Bake for 20–30 minutes or until a cake tester comes out clean. Cool and eat. Refrigerate leftovers.

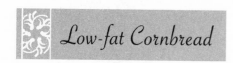

Low-fat Cornbread

A great bread alternative.

SERVES 9

NUTRITIONAL ANALYSIS: (SERVING SIZE ⅑ RECIPE) CALORIES 214 FAT 5G SAT FAT 0G
CHOLESTEROL 0MG PROTEIN 4G CARBOHYDRATE 25G FIBER 1G SODIUM 214MG

---

1 cup cornmeal

1 cup flour

2 Tbsp sugar

1 Tbsp baking powder

¼ tsp salt

2 egg whites

1 cup non-fat milk

3 Tbsp oil

Preheat oven to 375 degrees. Combine dry ingredients and mix well. Add egg whites, milk and oil. Stir until moistened. Pour into an 8x8-inch baking dish prepared with nonstick cooking spray. Bake for 20–25 minutes or until cake tester comes out clean.

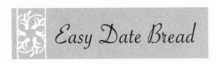

Easy Date Bread

*N*o one will guess that this delicious treat is fat-free! Serve it for breakfast, lunch or dinner.

SERVES 12

NUTRITIONAL ANALYSIS: (SERVING SIZE 1 SLICE) CALORIES 130 FAT 0.5G SAT FAT 0G
CHOLESTEROL 0MG PROTEIN 3G CARBOHYDRATE 30G FIBER 2G SODIUM 57MG

---

2 cups dates, chopped

1 tsp baking soda

1 cup hot water

2 egg whites

½ cup sugar

1 tsp vanilla extract

1½ cups flour

Preheat oven to 350 degrees. Place dates in a small bowl. Add baking soda to water and pour over dates. In a food processor, blend the egg whites, sugar and vanilla. Add about ¼ of the date/water mixture and process until fairly smooth. Add flour and process until blended. Add the remaining date/water mixture and process briefly for 15–30 seconds. Stir to be sure mixture is thoroughly blended. Pour into a 5x9-inch loaf pan prepared with nonstick spray. Bake for 60–75 minutes. Cool and slice. Can be served with non-fat cream cheese or ricotta.

Desserts

Everyday Banana Bread

Delicious and moist.

SERVES 10

NUTRITIONAL ANALYSIS: (SERVING SIZE ⅒ LOAF) CALORIES 156 FAT 3G SAT FAT 0G
CHOLESTEROL 0MG PROTEIN 3G CARBOHYDRATE 29G FIBER 1.5G SODIUM 243MG

---

3 ripe bananas, mashed

2 egg whites

2 Tbsp canola oil

⅓–½ cup sugar

¼ cup non-fat milk

½ tsp salt

½ tsp baking soda

1 tsp baking powder

1½ cups flour

Preheat oven to 350 degrees. In a large mixing bowl, combine the first five ingredients and blend well. Gently blend in the dry ingredients and stir until moistened. Pour into a 5x9-inch loaf pan coated with nonstick cooking spray. Bake for 50–55 minutes, until a knife comes out clean. Refrigerate leftovers.

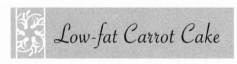

Low-fat Carrot Cake

Healthful and delicious. Make half the recipe in an 8x8–inch pan for a smaller gathering.

SERVES 18

NUTRITIONAL ANALYSIS: (SERVING SIZE ⅟₁₈ OF CAKE) CALORIES 172 FAT 4G SAT FAT 0G
CHOLESTEROL 0MG PROTEIN 3G CARBOHYDRATE 31G FIBER 2G SODIUM 145MG

---

4 cups shredded carrots (not packed)

8-oz can crushed pineapple in its own juice

1½ cups sugar

4 egg whites

1 cup white flour

1 cup whole wheat flour

⅓ cup oil

2 tsp vanilla

2 tsp baking soda

2 tsp cinnamon

1 tsp allspice

¼ tsp salt

½ cup raisins (yellow or black, as desired)

Preheat oven to 375 degrees. Mix all ingredients together and pour into a 13x9–inch pan prepared with nonstick cooking spray. Bake for 30–40 minutes or until cake tester inserted in center comes out clean. Cool and cut into 18 servings. Refrigerate leftovers.

Acknowledgments

While my guru's Integral Yoga teachings formed the theoretical thread and practical applications for *Dr. Yoga,* it took an international coalition to produce and assist me in writing it. An extraordinary team of distinguished mentors, colleagues, friends, associates, and relatives contributed their time, expertise, inspiration, and support, directly and indirectly, to both the creative and scientific process that produced the end result.

First and foremost I want to respectfully acknowledge and express my appreciation to the internationally renowned Penguin Group for publishing this book. My sincere thanks to the distinguished Jeremy Tarcher, founder of the Penguin Group's Tarcher imprint, for inviting me to write a book that would document the pioneering ways in which yoga is being used in the mainstream medical community. I was privileged to have his editorial guidance from the inception through my manuscript's early developmental stages.

Respectful gratitude to the dynamic publisher of the Tarcher imprint, Joel Fotinos, whose vision, faith, generosity, and support of every aspect of this project smoothed the way to writing it. Heartfelt gratitude to my editor, the incomparable Sara Carder, who shepherded it through all of its rigorous incarnations, for her enduring guidance and support. Her professional insights were invaluable in guiding and inspiring its execution every step of the way.

I was extraordinarily blessed and privileged to have the foundational and professional advice and wise counsel of my London and New York agents, Liz Puttick and Joelle Delbourgo, who tirelessly advocated on my behalf. They each helped to steer my book strategically from the business and developmental process through some tense moments to the final stages of publication. Throughout this process, I was also extremely fortunate to have the astute editorial assistance of Barbara Vesey, a London-based author and editor, who helped me to polish and transform my material into its final form.

My enduring gratitude to the renowned Dean Ornish, M.D., whom I am privileged to regard as both a dear friend and colleague, for his continued support and endorsement of my work through years as his referral therapist and for generously offering to provide the foreword for my book. Along with so many other medical professionals, I am indebted to him for breaking ground and creating medical history with his scientific exploration and application of Integral Yoga through his best-selling book and program on reversing heart disease. One of Sri Swami Satchidananda's most internationally acclaimed and influencial devotees, Dean serves as a constant inspiration and role model to me of what is possible.

I am also profoundly appreciative and honored by the association that I have with Cedars-Sinai Medical Center's Preventive and Rehabilitative Center (PRCC) as their Hatha Yoga Cardiac Therapist. It was this valued association with Cedars-Sinai that inspired the invitation to write this book. Thank you to the PRCC's medical director, the renowned and distinguished C. Noel Bairey Merz, M.D., with whom I have the amazing privilege of working. Words can't express my gratitude for her continued endorsement and support of my work there, and for so graciously offering to provide the preface for my book. My sincere thanks also to our associate director, Donna Polk, M.D., and Richard Gordon, M.A., patient program director, for their inspiration and constant advocacy of my work. My respectful appreciation to the rest of the PRCC medical and administrative staff whose tireless dedication to providing the most outstanding and innovative patient care available is also a continued source of inspiration to me.

Special thanks to Mary Felando, nutritionist for the PRCC, who graciously accepted my invitation to write the nutritional component for my book. I am grateful for her collaboration and support.

Respectful appreciation to P. K. Shah, M.D., director of cardiology at Cedars-Sinai Medical Center, for graciously offering to contribute his distinguished endorsement to my book. In the clinical and research aspects of my book I was also privileged to work with and have the medical expertise of some of the most respected medical dignitaries and researchers in their field. Sandra (Amrita) McLanahan, M.D., author of *Alternatives to Surgery,* provided clinical commentary while also contributing invaluable detailed medical research and documentation. I wish to gratefully acknowlege the eminent Herbert Benson, M.D., Andrew Weil, M.D., and Deepak Chopra, M.D., for their resource material and for continuing to serve as courageous role models for those of us in the medical community.

Adam Skolnick, featured writer for *LA Yoga* magazine, was also invaluable in contributing to my book's medical authenticity by vetting physicians throughout the United States and distilling clinical verifications of the medical uses of yoga. Special thanks also to the distinguished Dr. Sharma in India, and Michael Boda, Ph.D., Washington, D.C., for additional invaluable research contributions.

Thank you to David Kearney, OMD, who during my clinical internship served as my primary mentor. I'm deeply grateful for all he has contributed to my growth as a clinical medical practitioner as well as to my book. Sincere thanks to Ken Desure, D.C., and Gary Jacobs, D.C., for their support of my yoga and therapy practice, which also helped to provide the practical clinical foundation for my book. Special thanks to Leslie Bogart, R.N., a highly regarded and respected yoga teacher and therapist, for contributing her own professional clinical insights, experience and patient testimonies to my book. Special thanks also to the invaluable contributions of the distinguished oncologist Dwight McKee, M.D., the distinguished Steven Pacia, M.D., and Trisha Spoto of the NYU Epilepsy Center, Deborah Mulnick, R.N., and Jnani Chapman, R.N., of University of San Francisco Medical Center.

My sincere and heartfelt thanks to my extended professional family, Stephanie Hurcost, Buffy Ford Stewart, Lindsay Crouse, Ed and Debbie Shapiro, John Stewart, Bonnie Reiss, Jerry, Janet and Katie Zucker, Diane Ladd, Pia Zadora, Kadie

Riklis, Laura Dern, Judith Paige Mitchell, Woody and Noreen Fraser, Gary Bart, Willa Mamet and Zasha Mamet, Barnett Kellman and Nancy Mehta Kellman, Annie Appleby, and to my nephew Michel Moisant.

Grateful appreciation to Wendy and Amanda Goldberg, Hal Cooper, Buffy Ford Stewart, and Luke Stewart for serving as yoga models for my book and to Lindsay Crouse for generously offering her home as a location for our photo shoot. Very special thanks to Wendy Goldberg for her assistance in holding the book's photography to the highest industry standard and for her personal and professional support.

I'm deeply grateful to Anna Rottenberg, Howard Rutman, and all of my cardiac patients at Cedars-Sinai Medical Center and to my private patients, including SMT and Kory Tatyaran, for contributing their inspiring personal testimonies of how yoga has been effective as a clinical modality in the treatment of medical conditions.

Through the years, I have been privileged to provide therapy to some of the most respected legends and dignitaries of our time in the film, TV and music industries. I would like to thank in particular Candice Bergen, Jane Fonda, Diane Ladd, Angela Lansbury, Laura Dern, Jeff Goldblum, Oliver Stone, Marlo Thomas, Sally Kirkland, and B.D.

Grateful acknowledgments to my personal family members, Judy and Bill Moisant, Jean-David, Angie and Kohl Moisant; and Betty, Adolph, Rosie and Steven Waedelich for their love and support; and to my parents, John and Alice Heriza, in loving and grateful memory.

Grateful acknowlegments to my early mentors at Immaculate Heart College, Sister Lenore Dowling, Ph.D., Sister Margaret Rose, Ph.D., and Sister Ruth Marie Gibbons, Ph.D., who served as role models for stretching beyond boundaries, change and growth. Thank you to award-winning writer Megan Terry for first introducing me to the enlightened possibilities of the creative process through yoga. My enduring appreciation to her for her generous support and confidence in me, both professionally and personally, which made a critical difference in my life.

Special thanks to my additional extended family; the members of the Integral Yoga Teaching Center in Los Angeles; the distinguished Sri Murugesh Gounder, director of the Toronto Integral Yoga Teaching Center, his wife Aruna and daughter Sheela, and to Swami Asokananda, Swami Chidananda, Swami Ramananda, Swami Karunananda and all of the monastics and members of Satchidananda Ashram who contributed support and inspiration for my book. Heartfelt gratitude to Amma Kidd for her enduring encouragement. Respectful thanks to D. R. Kaarthikeyan, Esq., distinguished senior representative of H.H. Sri Swami Satchidananda and former director of the Central Bureau of Investigation and Director General of the National Human Rights Commission, for his valued contributions to my book and for his inspiration and prayers, and to Ramaswamy Gounder, president of Integral Yoga Institute, India.

Special acknowledgment of all of the members of Integral Yoga International organization for their enduring dedication to the legacy and teachings of our revered guru, and to Alice Coltrane (Swami Turiyasangitananda), Peter Max, Carole King, Tara Guber and the Harilela family.

Respectful acknowlegment of and grateful appreciation to the President's Council on Physical Fitness and Sports, with special thanks to the distinguished executive director, Melissa Johnson, and to Christine Spain and Janice Meer.

Grateful appreciation to renowned photographer Art Streiber for his signature photography. Special thanks to Vonetta at Montage, director of production, Hugh, Anna and everyone at at Digital Fusion, Smashbox Studio, Phillip Carreon and Brian at Estilo Hair Salon and to Byron Hair and Makeup Studio.

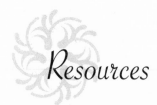

Resources

Recommended reading

YOGA AND MEDITATION

Selected Books by Sri Swami Satchidananda
Integral Yoga Hatha
To Know Your Self
Beyond Words
The Healthy Vegetarian
The Golden Present
The Yoga Sutras of Patanjali

Videotapes

Yoga with a Master (Hatha Yoga video recommended by Cedars-Sinai Preventive and Rehabilitative Cardiac Center)

Spiritual Help for Addictions

AIDS and Other Illness: Finding Hope in a Time of Crisis

Healing with Yoga

Johns Hopkins Medical School: Lecture on alternatives to conventional medicine

Meditation: The Path to Happiness

Freedom

Essential Teachings for Life

Yoga for Children

Audiotapes and CDs

Guided Relaxation and Affirmations for Inner Peace (recommended by Cedars-Sinai Preventive and Rehabilitative Cardiac Center)

Natural Health, Natural Medicine

Spontaneous Healing

Deepak Chopra, M.D.

Ageless Body, Timeless Mind

Seven Spiritual Laws of Success

Perfect Digestion

Quantum Healing

Janet Travell, M.D., and David G. Simons, M.D.

Myofascial Pain and Dysfunction

The Trigger Point Manual: Volumes I and II

Other Recommended Yoga Books

Sri Swami Satchidananda: Apostle of Peace (Sita Bordow)

Lotus Prayer Book (Swami Karunananda)

Imagine That (Kenneth Cohen)

Sparkling Together (Jyothi Ma)

Unconditional Love (Ed and Deb Shapiro)

Yoga: The Poetry of the Body (Rodney Yee)

Guided Meditation—Basic Techniques

The Breath of Life—Level I (Integral Yoga Pranayama I)

The Breath of Life—Level II

Holistic Health and Yoga

Trust and Faith

Selected Books by Sri Swami Sivananda

Concentration and Meditation

Mind—Its Mysteries and Control

Yoga in Daily Life

Sure Ways to Success in Life and God-Realization

Health and Hatha Yoga

What Becomes of the Soul After Death

MEDICINE/HOLISTIC HEALTH

Dean Ornish, M.D.

Dr. Dean Ornish's Program for Reversing Heart Disease

Eat More, Weigh Less

Love and Survival

Sandra McLanahan, M.D., and David McLanahan, M.D.

Surgery and Its Alternatives: How to Make the Right Choices for Your Health

Andrew Weil, M.D.

Spontaneous Healing

8 Weeks to Optimum Health

Health and Healing

Yoga for Wellness (Gary Kraftsow)

The Woman's Book of Yoga and Health (Linda Sparrowe)

Yoga Rx (Larry Payne)

For a comprehensive selection of other yoga and alternative health–related books and audio/DVD/video products by H.H. Sri Swami Satchidananda, H.H. Sri Swami Sivananda, and various other authors, access Integral Yoga Distribution at www.yogahealthbooks.com.

INTEGRAL YOGA

Satchidananda Ashram-Yogaville
Information on guest stays, yoga and yoga training programs
www.yogaville.org

Integral Yoga Magazine
www.iymagazine.org

Integral Yoga Teachers Association
(to locate an Integral Yoga teacher in your area)
www.iyta.org

The official Sri Swami Satchidananda website
Information on the life and teachings of Sri Swami Satchidananda
www.satchidananda.org

Integral Yoga Institute of New York
www.integralyogany.org

Integral Yoga Institute of San Francisco
www.integralyogasf.org

www.iycenter.com

INTEGRATIVE MEDICINE

Without some kind of medical compass, it can be very confusing to know where or even how to begin looking for a reliable medical resource option. When confronted with a serious condition or even for routine health care, particularly when considering a more holistic alternative or adjunct to conventional medicine, the search can be daunting. The following is a list of renowned, reliable and easily accessible complementary medical resources considered by professionals in the medical mainstream to set the highest standard in integrative medicine today.

Cedars-Sinai Medical Center
C. Noel Bairey, M.D.
Director of the Preventive and Rehabilitative Cardiac Center; Holder of the Chair in Woman's Health, Medical Director of Women's Health

Donna Polk, M.D., MPH
Assistant Medical Director, Cedars-Sinai Preventive and Rehabilitive Cardiac Center

Nirmala Heriza, B.A., CYT
Hatha Yoga Cardiac Therapist, Cedars-Sinai Preventive and Rehabilitive Cardiac Center; President, Integral Yoga Center of Los Angeles; President, United Council on Yoga, a partner of the President's Council on Physical Fitness and Sports for the President's Challenge Programs
www.cshs.org

Preventive Medicine Research Institute
Founder/President/Director: Dean Ornish, M.D., Cardiology
www.pmri.org

Mayo Clinic
www.mayoclinic.org

National Center for Complementary and Alternative Medicine
www.nccam.org

The Ayurvedic Institute
President: Dr. Vasant Lad
www.ayurveda.com

Andrew Weil, M.D.
www.drweil.com

Deepak Chopra, M.D.
www.chopra.com

Commonweal Cancer Help Programs
President, Michael Lerner, Ph.D.
www.commonweal.org

Carolinas Integrative Health Center
Medical Director: Russ Greenfield, M.D.
www.carolinas.org/services/

Robert F. Spetzler, M.D., Neurology
www.bnaneuro.net/

Mehmet Oz, M.D., Cardiology
New York Columbia Presbyterian Hospital
www.columbiasurgery.org

Herbert Benson, M.D., Cardiology
Mind-Body Medical Institute
www.mbmi.org/

Steven Pacia, M.D., Neurology
Trish Spoto, Program Director
NYU Comprehensive Epilepsy Center
www.nyuepilepsy.org

Himalayan Institute for Yoga Science and Philosophy
www.himalayaninstitute.org/

Research Group for Mind Body Dynamics
Obsessive Compulsive Disorders
www.theinternetyogi.com/

Kundalini Yoga and Insomnia
Sat Bir Singh, M.D., Harvard scientist
Khalsa@hms.harvard.edu

UCLA Pain Pediatrics Center for depression and chronic pain
Lonnie Zeltzer, M.D.
www.healthcare.ucla.edu

Canyon Ranch Retreat Center
Mark Hyman, Medical Director of Canyon Ranch in the Berkshires
Yoga for Addiction
www.canyonranch.com

Stanford Center for Integrative Medicine
Combines conventional and complementary medical modalities including yoga in the treatment of acute and chronic disease.
Dr. David Spiegel, Medical Director
www.stanfordhospital.com

University of Wisconsin Center for Integrative Medicine
Combines conventional and complementary medical modalities including yoga in the treatment of acute and chronic disease.
David Rakel, M.D.
www.uwhospital.org

Duke Center for Integrative Medicine
Combines conventional and complimentary medical modalities including yoga therapy for treatment of acute and chronic disease.
www.dukehealth.org

Medical Acupuncture Resources
www.medicalacupuncture.org

David Kearney, O.M.D.
www.powerhealing.com

N. Clare Heriza, M.D., MPH, DABMA
Specialty: Family Practice
Baker City, OR 97814
Phone: (541) 524-9490
Fax: (541) 524-9491

Yoga- and Health-Related Publications and Products

Integral Yoga Distribution

www.yogahealthbooks.com

www.gaiam.com

www.yogainternational.com

www.yogajournal.com

www.adamskolnick.com

www.layogamagazine.com

www.yogaforce.com

Yoga- and Health-Related Websites

www.webmd.com

www.holistic-online.com

www.yogasite.com

www.yogakids.com

Yoga Facilities

www.yogaalliance.com

www.bikramyoga.com

Other Distinguished Health-Related Referrals

President's Council on Physical Fitness and Sports/President's Challenge Programs
www.fitness.gov
Executive Director: Melissa Johnson

United Council on Yoga (UCY)
President: Nirmala Heriza
www.presidentschallenge.org
(To access UCY: 1. click advocates 2. click nonprofit on left menu bar.)

The Larry King Cardiac Foundation
A nonprofit organization created to provide funding for heart bypass operations and heart transplants for individuals with limited means and inadequate insurance.
www.lkcf.org

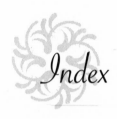

Index

About the Author

NIRMALA HERIZA is a Hatha yoga cardiac therapist at Cedars-Sinai Medical Center Preventive and Rehabilitative Cardiac Center. President of the United Yoga Council and director of the Los Angeles Integral Yoga® Center, she is a senior disciple of the renowned yoga master and founder of Integral Yoga, H.H. Sri Swami Satchidananda. Heriza also has a private yoga therapy practice in Los Angeles that serves many celebrities in the film, television, and music industries.

About the Contributors

SANDRA MCLANAHAN, M.D., the medical consultant for *Dr. Yoga*, is a family physician and executive medical director of the Integral Health Center in Buckingham, Virginia. Coauthor of *Surgery and Its Alternatives*, she lives in Buckingham, Virginia.

ADAM SKOLNICK is a freelance journalist in the health/travel field who was a principal contributing medical researcher for *Dr. Yoga*. He writes for such national publications as *Outside, Islands, Spa, Yoga International, LA Weekly,* and *LA Yoga,* a weekly yoga magazine that he also helped launch. Other credits include the forthcoming book *Ordinary Buddhas* and an independent film in progress. Visit his website at www.adamskolnick.com.